The SIMPLYRAW KITCHEN

Dearest Sylheia,

Health is not everything — but without Health everything is nothing.

Remembering the good times together and much love,

Alse

The SIMPLY*RAW* KITCHEN

plant-powered, gluten-free, and mostly raw recipes for healthy living

Natasha Kyssa

with **Ilse Kyssa**

Arsenal Pulp Press 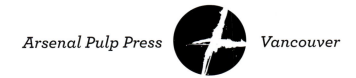 Vancouver

THE SIMPLYRAW KITCHEN
Copyright © 2013 by Natasha Kyssa

SECOND PRINTING: 2014

ARSENAL PULP PRESS
Suite 202 – 211 East Georgia St.
Vancouver, BC V6A 1Z6
Canada
arsenalpulp.com

The publisher gratefully acknowledges the support of the Government of Canada (through the Canada Book Fund) and the Government of British Columbia (through the Book Publishing Tax Credit Program) for its publishing activities.

The author and publisher assert that the information contained in this book is true and complete to the best of their knowledge. All recommendations are made without the guarantee on the part of the author and publisher. The author and publisher disclaim any liability in connection with the use of this information. For more information, contact the publisher.

Note for our UK readers: measurements for non-liquids are for volume, not weight.

Design by Gerilee McBride
Cover and interior photographs by Trevor Lush
Editing by Susan Safyan
Sprouts and microgreens photographed for this book courtesy of Butterfly Sky Farms

Printed and bound in Canada

Library and Archives Canada Cataloguing in Publication

Kyssa, Natasha, 1961-, author
    The SimplyRaw kitchen : plant-powered, gluten-free, and mostly raw recipes for healthy living / Natasha Kyssa.

 Includes index.
 Issued in print and electronic formats.
 ISBN 978-1-55152-505-1 (pbk.).—ISBN 978-1-55152-506-8 (epub)

    1. Raw foods. 2. Cooking (Natural foods). 3. Vegan cooking.
4. Gluten-free diet—Recipes. 5. Cookbooks. I. Title.

TX837.K97 2013   641.5'636   C2013-903241-X
                                            C2013-903242-8

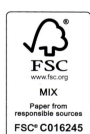

DEDICATION

To my dearest mother Ilse, who has had the most extraordinary influence on my life. You are an inspiration to me and to all who know you.

And to Ann Wigmore, whose vision sparked mine.

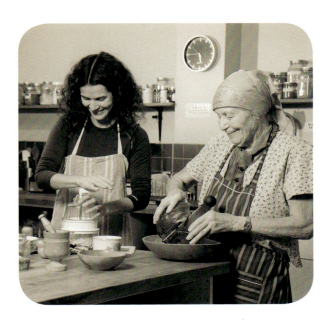

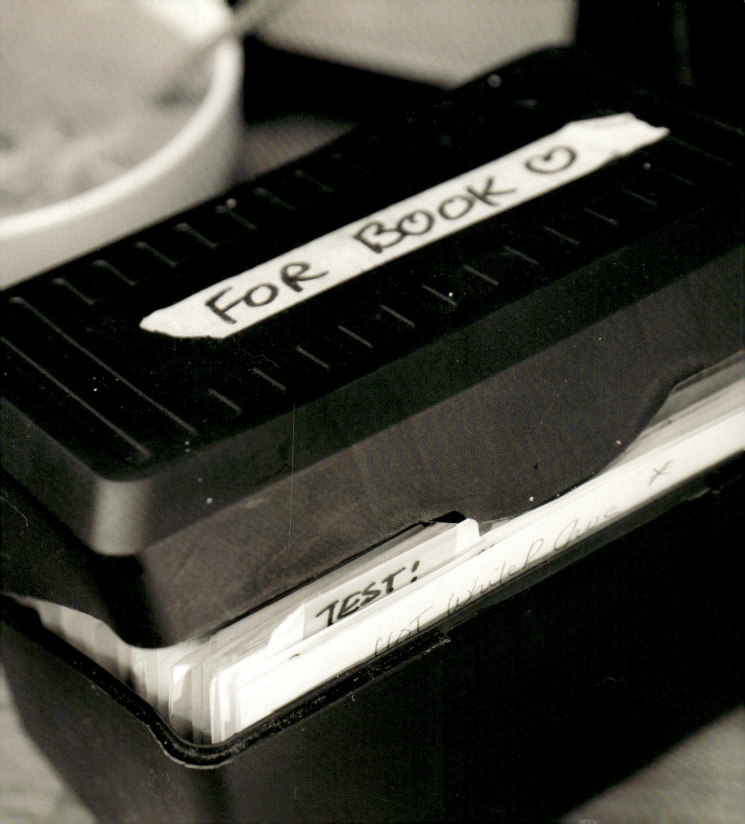

CONTENTS

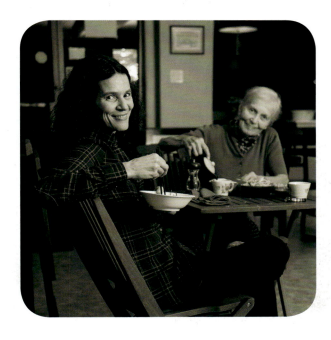

Foreword by Richard Anderson   9

Introduction   11

A Mother's Blessing by Ilse Kyssa   15

The Whole Foods Approach to Going Raw   17

Kitchen Essentials   23

The Ingredients   28

The Tools   33

The Techniques   36

Key to Symbols   47

Beverages   49

Breakfasts   71

Soups   81

Salads & Salad Dressings   105

Pâtés, Dips, Spreads & Cheezes   127

Mains   147

Desserts & Sweet Treats   177

Acknowledgments   201

Index   203

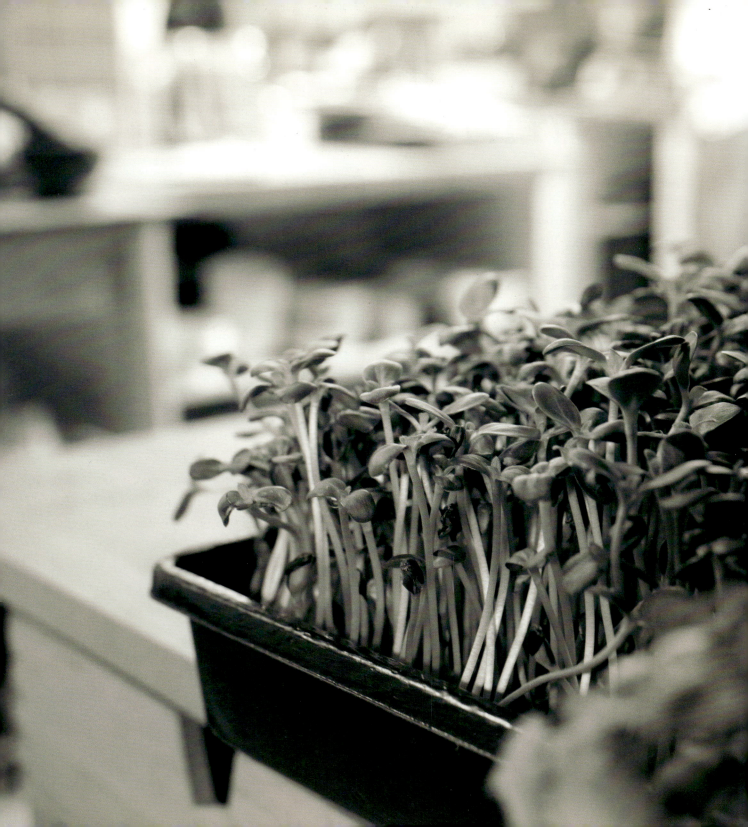

FOREWORD

Richard Anderson

In the fall of 1976, I attended a seminar presented by a Seattle-based cancer organization which had brought together from around the world doctors who had an average success rate in treating cancer *four times greater* than most oncologists; Dr Bernard Jensen's and Dr John Christopher's success rates, for example, were over seventy percent, while Dr William Kelly's was ninety-three percent. These statistics were verified by the Sloan Kettering Foundation.

What I learned that day changed my life.

After the seminar, I decided to find out just how effective these doctors really were—and if they were really that good, then I wanted to know what they did to produce such incredible results. First, I discovered that these physicians were not only specialists in treating cancer, but were also able to heal other health problems. As well, I learned that most of the patients came to them after they had tried conventional therapies and met with undesirable results; the patients were considered difficult cases—and still, these doctors achieved unprecedented success.

Dr Jensen, for example, had the highest success rate for treating leukemia in America— forty percent— when most medical doctors were close to zero. Jensen told me that he had first learned his unusual healing techniques from other doctors who had reported success, and then he set out to improve upon what they had done. I decided to do the same.

Each of these exceptional doctors broke away from the status quo of modern medicine and studied alternative philosophies and treatments. Their theories and treatments were vastly different from what most medical doctors believed and did, even though many of them *were* medical doctors themselves. First, they all treated causes, not just symptoms. Second, not one of them believed in the germ theory that is taught in allopathic medical schools. Third, with very few exceptions, they never used drugs, which they considered to be toxic and thus interfered with true healing. Fourth, all of them put their patients on some form of deep cleansing program. And last but most important, they all put their patients on healthy diets, that is, on alkaline-forming vegetarian regimens.

After many years of studying the philosophies and methods of treatments of Drs Jenson, Christopher, Kelly, and others who had consistent and unusual success, I discovered that they all shared the same view as to the root of most health problems, excluding physical injuries: toxins and acids, as well as nutritional deficiencies. Further, negative thoughts and emotions that had become stored in the subconscious were creating and sustaining harmful patterns, habits, and addictions.

But where are all these toxins and acids coming from? We breathe many toxins into our bodies and absorb them through the skin—more so now than at any other time in history—but the vast majority of toxins and acids come from the food we eat.

The Standard American Diet is a toxic and acidifying diet. It is the number-one cause of almost all health problems we currently face. Why is the human animal plagued with so many preventable illnesses such as cancer and heart disease? Humans are the only mammals who cook their food, the only mammals who drink other animals' milk, and the only mammals who continue to drink milk after being weaned. If we were designed to be meat-eating animals, then we would have to eat it like other meat-eating animals do—raw, guts first, and including blood, skin, fur, and bones, for these are the only alkaline tissues. Animals that eat only muscle, like humans, become sick.

The most difficult problem people encounter as they try to shift away from the Standard American Diet is dealing with their addictions to familiar foods.

When they begin to eat the foods that are natural to humans—i.e., raw fruits and vegetables—they miss their old meals. What has long been needed is a book that teaches people the fundamentals of eating healthfully, along with recipes that are easy to prepare and taste delicious. I know many vegetarians who do not eat healthfully because they simply do not know how to make their food taste good. *The SimplyRaw Kitchen* solves all these problems.

This book is rich in wisdom, and inspires us to move forward into greater health, energy, and enjoyment in eating and living. Natasha understands what the vast majority of conventional medical doctors have neglected, and she provides readers with recipes that will allow them to live and eat vibrantly and healthfully.

By following the suggestions in *The SimplyRaw Kitchen*, you too will achieve excellent health and a longer, happier life.

Richard Anderson, ND, NMD, is the author of Cleanse & Purify Thyself *and founder of Arise and Shine.*

INTRODUCTION

The SimplyRaw Kitchen was written to inspire you to include fresh, whole, nutrient-rich foods in your diet in a balanced and loving way and to experience just how extraordinarily delicious healthy eating can be. Eating whole plant foods is a tasty way to fuel your body with an abundance of essential vitamins, minerals, enzymes, and phytonutrients. The key to enjoying a healthy plant-based diet, as with any diet, is to eat a wide variety of foods and to have a range of simple recipes that use basic ingredients and take little time and effort to prepare.

The life-giving recipes in this book are 100-percent vegan, 100-percent gluten-free, and almost all of them raw. Over many years of testing, tasting, and experimenting, I created these recipes to encourage you to enjoy making meals in your own kitchen for lifelong health. All of them are delicious and provide optimal nutrition from fresh whole plant foods, filling your body with energy and vitality; I'm confident that you will want to enjoy them on a regular basis. I wrote this book with my mother Ilse; we spent many spirited hours together in the kitchen fine-tuning her recipes, which are comprised of tasty contemporary versions of traditional Eastern European comfort foods that are—wait for it—cooked. While I am a strong advocate of the healing and nutritional power

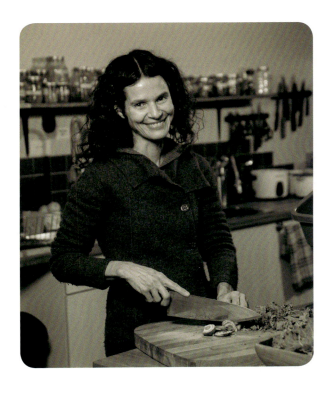

of raw foods, I also understand the challenges of a fully raw diet. As well, over the years, I've seen many people struggle when they switch to a healthy eating regimen overnight. Sometimes the best approach is to transition gradually to a new diet, a process that may include cooked foods—slowly replacing unhealthy meal choices with healthier ones until the habit becomes ingrained. *The SimplyRaw Kitchen* is filled with practical tips and advice on transitioning to a raw diet, along with a few nostalgic Austrian tales interwoven with fascinating stories and facts about plants and their healing properties.

My SimplyRaw Journey

My traditional Eastern European family was noticeably different from others in our neighborhood: my parents spoke Russian and German at home, we listened and danced to lively Turkish folk music in front of an open fire, and I went (reluctantly) to Russian Sunday school. Unlike the other children we knew, we wore second-hand clothes, and we were the only family that had a compost heap in the backyard for kitchen scraps. And unlike many women in the 1970s, my Austrian mother stayed at home to look after our family. She worked selflessly—cooking, baking, mending, ironing, nurturing—and always put the needs of her husband and children first.

We didn't eat the typical North American diet, either. Meals were simple and always prepared from scratch using natural, fresh ingredients—often enhanced by my mother's penchant for herbs. Delicious salads, homemade borscht, sauerkraut, and stuffed cabbage rolls were my childhood favorites. Whether we wanted to or not, we sat down as a family at every meal, with my father, the patriarch, at the head of the table, where he was always served first. As a teenager, I was embarrassed about my home life and avoided bringing friends over after school. I envied friends who were allowed to eat white bread, canned soups, ice cream, potato chips, and other "normal" foods.

And yet, I found refuge in my mother's warm kitchen, often doing homework with the enticing aromas of her cooking enveloping me. I gradually became interested in flavorful world cuisine and started to create my own recipes, once winning the local community baking contest with my onion bread. I also began to discover my own dietary preferences—I was an animal lover and adopted a vegetarian diet. Soon after leaving home at the age of nineteen, I started my career as a fashion model propelling me to an exciting, glamorous life, in which I traveled to all parts of the globe and got paid ridiculous amounts of money to wear the latest fashions. After seven intense years, however, the pressures of having to maintain a size-zero body took its toll. Like many models in the industry, I experimented with every diet imaginable in a desperate attempt to stay thin—with little success. This led to an eating disorder and a dangerous, unhealthy life of addictions to alcohol, tobacco, prescription drugs, caffeine, and processed foods.

In 1990, when I was twenty-nine, my health declined to a disturbing low: I was exhausted, depressed, socially withdrawn, and my weight regularly fluctuated by more than forty pounds (18 kg). It was hardly the glamorous life that most people imagine fashion models enjoying. It was at this low point that my personal journey to health began. In a moment of clarity, I realized how far I had strayed from the natural whole foods on which I had been raised. I slowly cleaned up my diet, shifting away from toxic, synthetic, and chemically laden foods and toward simple, unprocessed plant-based meals such as salads, lightly steamed vegetables, and cooked broths and soups. Not surprisingly, my health took a dramatic turn for the better: my depression diminished, I had more energy, my weight normalized, my complexion improved, my hair got shinier and, most rewarding of all, I was able to resolve many of the personal issues that had caused me to make poor food choices in the first place. The closer I ate to nature, the better I felt. It was that simple.

> *Watch my TEDx talk online, "TEDxOttawa, Natasha Kyssa, Let Food Be Thy Medicine," **www.youtube.com/watch?v=rlFuFl44c5Y**, to view my raw foods story.*

Within a few years, I had become a 100-percent raw foodist, fueling my body with fresh uncooked fruits, vegetables, nuts, seeds, and legumes. As my personal journey evolved, I came to understand first-hand that food is indeed powerful—what we eat can transform our bodies and emotions, our health and our spirit. I am certain that I would not be here today had I not taken responsibility for my health and changed my self-destructive ways.

Paradoxically, despite the fact that medical research has advanced phenomenally over the last century, and we have learned much about the impact of good health and nutrition, more people than ever are struggling with health challenges, many of them severe or life-threatening. Most North Americans today accept degenerative chronic conditions and diseases—including obesity, diabetes, atherosclerosis, heart disease, osteoporosis, cancer, and depression—as part of the normal aging process. Digestive issues, allergies, and other food sensitivities (such as celiac disease) are also a growing problem for many people. It is clear to me and many others that these health concerns are directly related to our deviation from a natural, whole foods diet.

Today's food is very different from that of our ancestors. The natural staples that our foremothers ate have been replaced with instant, pre-packaged, low-nutrient, high-caloric overly processed "un-foods," and non-organic fruits and vegetables grown with the help of carcinogenic chemicals (such as pesticides, fungicides, and herbicides). Food is picked unripe and out of season, shipped long distances, and has a ridiculously long shelf life thanks to the never-ending list of preservatives and additives. There is no question that food affects our health. But food is no longer simply fuel; it has become a social act. Every time we eat something, we are making environmental, ecological, and political choices. Whenever we sit down for a meal, we are supporting a food system that has serious effects on the earth's sustainability. We must regain our personal connection to our food. Over the past two decades, I have been blessed with the opportunity to show thousands of people around the world a simple yet powerful, nutrient-dense way of eating through my passion and business, SimplyRaw (*simplyraw.ca*), by teaching nutritional and cleansing programs and culinary workshops, and through my first book *The SimplyRaw Living Foods Detox Manual*. I am committed to my life's mission of spreading health one meal at a time through SimplyRaw Express, a restaurant in Ottawa, Canada, that I co-own and operate. And, along the way, I have witnessed some truly remarkable transformations in people who simply, yet profoundly, changed their diets.

The following recipes, which include both raw and cooked dishes, use the most wholesome ingredients available—real food, for real life! I hope I inspire you to approach healthy eating with long-lasting enthusiasm and balance. Whether you opt for an all-raw or cooked whole foods vegan diet, or a balance between the two, there's something here for everyone. I am grateful to be able to share with you the incredible joys of eating health-giving foods at each and every meal.

From my kitchen to yours, in health and gratitude,
Natasha

A MOTHER'S BLESSING

BY ILSE KYSSA

Few things bring us back to our childhood memories like food. When I was a child in Austria, we had to make do with what was grown in the countryside; these were the days before factory farming and artificially preserved foods. At home, the kitchen was the busiest room in the house, our favorite spot to gather, a place where everything was always full of life.

Grains, nuts, vegetables, and fruits came in their natural, unadulterated state. We grew fresh herbs in window boxes, hung apple slices on a cord from the kitchen ceiling to dry, shredded cabbage into a big barrel to ferment, and dried pumpkin seeds in the oven. We pickled and dried many foods and made jams and jellies without preservatives. We used rum and schnapps in tinctures and rubs; one of these, made with horse chestnuts soaked for six weeks in alcohol, was good for circulation when applied to the legs. In May of each year, we collected the delicate green buds from pine trees which, when mixed with honey, dissolved into a liquid. We then let them sit on a sunny window ledge, and after two months, we strained the liquid; this was how we made cough syrup. We appreciated the simple and natural tastes of unprocessed foods, free of chemical additives.

After I got married, I regularly cooked for my husband and our four children. We immigrated to

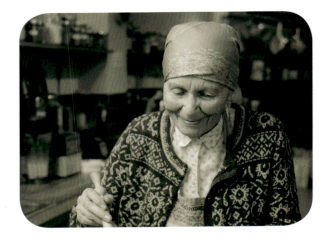

Canada in 1951. My husband liked to eat meat, but it was never a preference for me—not for health, but for moral reasons. In 1975, I started one of the first vegetarian tea rooms in Ottawa, called The Pantry. It was listed in *Ottawa Magazine* as a top spot for lunch and tea. Everything was made from scratch with mostly organic, local ingredients. Since I had no car, I did all the shopping by bicycle and took the kitchen scraps home for my garden compost. For my environmental efforts, I received the Whitton Award from the City of Ottawa in 1994. When I retired twenty years after opening the tea room, my dear friend Carolyn Best continued the tradition of serving wholesome, nutritious food there. In 2010, The Pantry celebrated its thirty-fifth anniversary.

In 2007, my daughter Natasha and I spent three weeks together at the Hippocrates Health Institute in Florida where we followed a raw foods diet (though I was allowed to eat a limited amount of steamed vegetables because of my age). Since then, I try to stay vegan and devote at least one day a week to eating raw. When Natasha asked me for vegan, gluten-free recipes from my own culinary background for this book, however, it was a challenge: Austrian cuisine is known for its meat-based dishes, creamy sauces, and rich, luscious pastries. I grew up eating Wiener Schnitzel and Apfelstrudel! I've reproduced some of my favorite recipes close to their original versions here, but adapted to be vegan and gluten-free. My dishes are simple, economical, and full of nutrient-rich ingredients.

Seasoning is very important. An old Austrian saying, "Not too little, not too much, is every good cook's special touch," is a good rule of thumb: use less seasoning to start, and add more after tasting. If you don't have an ingredient the recipe calls for, follow your instinct and substitute something similar, adding your own special touch.

I'd like to say a big thank you to Carolyn for always patiently answering my questions. Thank you, Jean-Paul St. Louis, for faithfully transcribing my often difficult-to-decipher handwriting and sending it to Natasha on the computer. Finally, special thanks to Natasha for her enthusiasm and encouragement and for reminding me that making food should be a joyful and relaxing experience. My mother used to say, "If you are not in the mood to sing—don't cook." I'm afraid that if we followed that saying, many of us would go hungry a lot of the time! I hope that you will enjoy yourself in the kitchen. Be creative. Stay healthy. And, last but not least, give gratitude for the food which gives us energy and nourishment.

Enjoy, and *Mahlzeit!*
Ilse

Note: *In the pages that follow, Ilse's stories are denoted by a light green arrow.*

THE WHOLE FOODS APPROACH TO GOING RAW

A whole food is any food in its most essential, pure, and basic form, its whole and natural state—a whole apple, a whole cucumber, a bean sprout, a kale leaf, a pineapple. Whole foods have not been processed, pasteurized, bottled, preserved, colored, canned, boxed, waxed, fumigated, injected with hormones or antibiotics, genetically modified, or irradiated. They don't contain additives or fillers. At their freshest, whole foods contain an abundance of vitamins, minerals, enzymes, and plant phytochemicals. These naturally occurring nutrients work together synergistically. Eating whole foods not only can make you feel better, they can prevent, and often even reverse, many diseases.

▶ *"Let food be thy medicine and medicine be thy food."* —Hippocrates, ca. 460–370 BCE

Think about how much time you devote to food every day—choosing, purchasing, storing, preparing, eating, digesting, assimilating, and absorbing it. Unfortunately, pre-packaged and fast foods are highly processed and filled with chemicals, refined sugars, artificial flavors, and saturated and trans-fats. These foods may be convenient but are completely lacking in vitamins, minerals, fiber, and nutrients that are essential to health.

Diabetes, heart disease, cancer, and other degenerative diseases are on the rise. But by eating more fresh vegetables, fruits, legumes, nuts, and seeds—that is, by providing our bodies with the key micronutrients that they need to function—we can prevent many illnesses. Current research shows a direct correlation between diet and health problems and supports the health benefits of plant-based diets; if you want to read more about this, I recommend *The China Study* by T. Colin Campbell (and see p. 25 for more titles).

While I believe that a raw vegan diet is essential for radiant health, I don't believe that there is one single dietary route for each and every person. Not only is our individual genetic makeup different from everyone else's, we also live in unique environments and have distinct needs. The food regimen that works well for one person may not be suitable for another. In fact, the eating habits that worked for you last year may no longer work for you now. However, there are basic universal principles around eating for optimal health that are applicable to almost everyone.

Here are some of them:

- Eat a plant-based diet. Plant-based foods are an excellent source of important vitamins, minerals, fiber, antioxidants, enzymes, and phytonutrients essential for optimal health. Many studies indicate that a plant-based diet that includes a good variety of different vegetables, fruits, sprouts, nuts, and seeds will provide all the nutrients required to support a healthy lifestyle.

- Eat fresh whole, unprocessed foods.
- Eat a high percentage of raw and fiber-rich foods.
- Eat organic foods.
- Eat ripe, in-season, and locally grown produce.
- Eat a variety of colorful fruits and vegetables to provide your body with a wide range of antioxidants and phytochemicals.
- Eat foods containing omega-3 fats.
- Eat mindfully.

Making the Transition to Raw

As a raw vegan for more than two decades, I remain deeply committed to this lifestyle. And while I believe whole-heartedly that a pure, raw, plant-based diet is the optimal way of eating, I've come to recognize that it's not easy for everyone to adopt or maintain. Over the many years that I've been involved in the field of health, I've met raw food enthusiasts, including friends, acquaintances, colleagues, staff, clients, and SimplyRaw Express customers, who were not able to sustain a 100-percent raw diet and who simply gave up and returned to the old habits that made them feel

unwell in the first place. I also noticed that they often felt guilty when they ate cooked foods, as if they'd committed a sin. I know only too well, as someone who's recovered from an eating disorder, that stressing about food or treating diet like a religion is unhealthy and counterproductive. It's healthier to consider your dietary habits as a transitional journey over time, to eat with joy, and to find a balance of food options that work well for your lifestyle. I do encourage you to move toward a raw vegan lifestyle, as the health benefits are phenomenal—but know that this journey can take years.

> *Not sure whether it's a fresh whole food or not? Ask yourself if you could have got it directly from nature—picked from a tree or a bush or dug from the soil—exactly as it is. If so, it's a whole food!*

Food nourishes us not only physically but emotionally, and eating is an experience connected to family, celebration, childhood memories, security, and love. Following a completely raw diet requires great effort, and socializing with family and friends who don't eat raw exclusively is by far the most challenging aspect, sometimes arousing feelings of isolation and deprivation. Living in a cold climate or having limited access to fresh foods can also present challenges.

Many raw foodists become so fixated on being all raw that they fall into the narrow mindset of "anything raw is better than anything cooked," and rely on nuts, seeds, oils, and other fats, which are hard to digest, especially when eaten in large amounts. Some also prefer the convenience of packaged raw food products (including so-called "superfoods") while forgoing the true superfoods: fresh fruits and vegetables. I believe that it is healthier to eat a clean, low-fat, plant-based diet consisting mostly of fresh raw produce, with a small amount of cooked whole foods (ideally eighty percent or more raw and no more than twenty-percent cooked) than to subsist on foods, raw or not, fabricated in a factory.

▶ *Real food doesn't come with labels!*

Including some cooked (but still vegan) recipes in this book provides a relaxed and manageable way to enjoy wholesome meals, without the challenge of eating all raw, all at once. For most people, dietary changes are best made gradually, replacing poor food choices with healthier versions, one meal at a time. To make the transition to a healthier lifestyle easier, and to help sustain it, gradually start including some of the cooked whole food recipes as replacements for unhealthier choices.

When I became a raw foodist in the early 1990s, there was no Internet—no websites or blogs, forums, or online support groups—no raw gurus or experts, raw cacao, "superfoods," or raw gourmet products. In many ways, it was easier then because there were

fewer conflicting messages. Inspirational pioneers such as Ann Wigmore, Norman Walker, Paavo Airola, Dr Richard Anderson, and Viktoras Kulvinskas all based their practices on fueling the human body with an abundance of vitamins, minerals, enzymes, and phytonutrients derived from fresh, whole, simple, and unprocessed plant foods.

▶ *Phytochemicals are chemical compounds that occur naturally in plants; they are biologically significant, but not considered essential nutrients. They do, however, have properties that help to protect us against disease. Raw fruits and vegetables are the best sources of phytochemicals.*

For me, raw veganism is a positive lifestyle centered on nourishment, compassion, flexibility, and love. This is why I have included some vegan versions of my old favorites from my mother's European kitchen—simple, whole food recipes free from animal products, gluten, or refined carbohydrates—to help you feel nourished on every level, at every meal. My approach is not about being 100-percent raw, but rather about being 100-percent healthy! This all-inclusive, health-focused approach is accessible to everyone: for those in transition; for raw foodists wanting to expand their repertoire; for those who wish to eat more healthy meals; and for those who, in the depth of winter, know that a warm bowl of hearty soup feeds the body, heart, and soul!

Good health is a holistic undertaking that requires proper nutrition, exercise, and the nurturing of our emotional, mental, and spiritual needs.

I encourage you to follow your own path and begin to increase the number and variety of high-quality raw foods in your meals in a gentle, loving way. Take your time, breathe, experiment, and enjoy the ride—because it is a lifetime journey. While a fully raw diet is not for everyone, fresh fruits and vegetables bursting with flavor and nutrients are!

I don't consider myself a chef, but I do enjoy food that is flavorful, fresh, and relatively easy to make. I am known to take a few shortcuts in the kitchen because, frankly, long hours spent preparing overly complicated recipes is simply not my idea of fun. The recipes in this book feature easy-to-find whole ingredients, and most of them require the use of equipment no more exotic than a blender or food processor, knife or grater.

 Fresh is best:
Nutrients are the most plentiful in fruits and vegetables just after they've been harvested. Fresh, ripe foods taste better. Local foods are not only fresher, but they also have a smaller carbon footprint than imported ones.

Transitioning to a raw diet can be intimidating at first, so take it slowly. Start your raw journey simply by adding more raw foods to your daily diet. This might mean beginning the day with juice or a smoothie, having a salad for lunch, and something raw to accompany dinner. Try to include more raw foods than cooked with every meal, and remember that blending and juicing can help you consume higher amounts of live nutrients.

Here are some tips to help you on your journey:

- Start your mornings raw with a green smoothie or freshly pressed juice, followed by a piece or two of fresh fruit, if you're still hungry. This is by far the simplest way of incorporating more fresh raw foods, and it also sets a healthy tone for the day! If you're pressed for time in the mornings, fill your blender up with all the ingredients (except for frozen fruit, if you're using it) and store the blender in the refrigerator for use first thing in the morning.

- Include a salad (with lots of sprouts) with every meal.

- Eat a blended raw soup for dinner or before the rest of your evening meal.

- Snack on fresh fruit and raw veggies when hungry.

- When socializing, always (and I mean always) bring a private stash of foods to snack on when hunger hits. I like to carry with me apples, nori, dulse, pumpkin seeds, and dried apricots—a mix of crunchy, chewy, sweet, and salty flavors to please the palate.

- Find a few recipes that you really enjoy and prepare them in advance for the upcoming week, so that you'll be less inclined to reach for something less healthy when you're in a rush.

- If you're going out for dinner, be sure to eat something nourishing before you leave the house. I also recommend carrying dried fruits and other easy-to-transport foods with you to the restaurant to discreetly jazz up salads. Remember to balance your meals—so if you order something less than optimal, balance it with a healthy raw choice.

- Drink plenty of water. Often we eat when we're not hungry but actually thirsty. Sip on fresh purified water throughout the day. I like to add a teaspoon or two of spirulina, or another form of powdered algae to my water bottle to keep me nourished and balanced— especially when I'm traveling and can't always get fresh juices.

- Most important, be gentle and patient with yourself; our eating habits are deeply ingrained and we can't expect to change overnight.

Friends and Family

One thing that I've learned over the years is that eating habits are very personal, and people often become defensive if given unwanted advice. Getting friends and family on board with your new way of eating can be challenging. As much as you may want to see your loved ones improve their health, always remember that the only person you truly have control over is yourself. Stay focused on your own well-being. The best thing you can do is to be a good example of how a whole foods diet can improve health, appearance, and attitude. You may find that your friends and family will become curious about your way of life and, in turn, take some steps to join you in your quest for better health.

Of course, there are always healthy guidelines that you can (discreetly) follow at home. Keep it fun and non-threatening; your family may be resistant at first, but they will eventually develop a taste for healthful foods. Offer your children a daily assortment of fresh fruits, vegetables, and other finger foods, and ensure that they are cut up and peeled for easy access. Kids also love smoothies, which will give you a creative way to slip in nutritional extras such as hemp, chia, flax seeds, and leafy greens without them even noticing.

Community

One of the most important elements of a lifestyle transition is to have good community support. While there are many online sites that help to create a communal experience, nothing beats good old-fashioned human contact. Potlucks are a creative way to meet others who share your interests, values, and enthusiasm for healthy eating. They are a great way to establish relationships, build community, and provide a sense of family, support, and inclusion. Plus, they're fun!

If you can't find a local potluck in your neighborhood, host your own and invite new friends. You can also plan a block party on your street or a picnic in the park.

Exercise

You can have the best diet in the world, but if you don't exercise, you will not achieve optimal health.

The benefits of regular exercise are hard to ignore: it plays a preventative role against heart disease, high blood pressure, diabetes, osteoporosis, and depression. Exercise boosts our body's natural defenses against cold and flu viruses. It also promotes improved circulation, lung function, sleep, muscle tone, and flexibility, and contributes to a positive attitude. To quote my eighty-five-years-young mother, who still works four days a week, practices yoga every day, and is more flexible than most people half her age: "Resting is rusting!"

Mindful Eating

How we eat can be as important as what we eat. Often we are in such a rush that we don't take time to truly appreciate the food in front of us. When we pause and pay attention to our meal, we establish a connection to the growing, harvesting, preparing, and nurturing of the food that went into it. We become more mindful, and we enjoy each bite with gratitude. We also begin to notice how the food we eat affects us. Before eating, take a moment of silence to really appreciate the meal in front of you.

KITCHEN ESSENTIALS

In this chapter, I describe essential ingredients and basic tools and techniques for putting together a healthy, mostly raw kitchen. The secret to preparing flavorful food is to use high-quality ingredients. But before discussing them in detail, I'd like to share the six basic principles that form the basis of my whole foods approach to raw:

1. Eat a plant-based diet.
2. Choose whole foods.
3. Eat a high percentage of raw foods.
4. Eat organic foods.
5. Get locally grown food.
6. Go gluten-free.

1. Eat a Plant-Based Diet

> *"There is absolutely no nutrient, no protein, no vitamin, no mineral, that we know of, that can't be obtained from plant-based foods." —Michael Klaper, MD, author of* **Vegan Nutrition: Pure and Simple**

The single most important choice that you can make in your diet is to avoid the consumption of animals and animal byproducts. The largest, most powerful animals, including elephants, horses, gorillas, and hippopotamuses, rely only on plant foods for protein and complete nutrition. There is no shortage of research supporting the choice of a plant-based diet;

the vegan lifestyle is gaining credibility and popularity as more people become aware of its health and environmental benefits. Here are just a few of the many reasons to choose a plant-based diet:

- Health: Eating lower on the food chain helps reduce the risk of heart disease, diabetes, and various forms of cancer. Vegetarians and vegans also have lower rates of illness and death from a number of other degenerative diseases.
- Environment: Meat consumption plays a large role in deforestation, water pollution, and soil degradation. A plant-based diet can ease both the pressures on the environment (less land clearance for livestock) and on atmospheric gases. A plant-based diet is the best choice for a sustainable planet.
- Compassion: Food-production animals suffer greatly during their short lives, enduring horribly inhumane living conditions and painful deaths. Pigs, cows, chickens, and other domesticated animals can think and feel just like our pets.
- End world hunger: More than enough food is currently grown to feed every human being in the world, but a huge percentage of (usually genetically modified) grains, soybeans, and

corn are produced to feed animals—a process that is highly energy inefficient. Instead, those same crops could be grown organically and serve as food for people.

- Higher collective consciousness: Choosing a plant-based diet brings us increased awareness, empowering us to make more responsible and ethical choices throughout our lives.

The Protein Myth

The need for protein—how much and from what sources—is a widely debated topic and often the subject of heated discussions. Old belief systems (and propaganda from the meat, dairy, and egg industries) have led many people to believe that we must eat meat to get our daily protein requirements. The truth is, in our society, most people eat far too much protein. (Protein deficiencies generally occur in underdeveloped countries where people do not have access to a variety of foods. They suffer not just from a lack of protein, but from an overall deficiency of calories and nutrients.)

Proteins are made up of chains of amino acids, which are the building blocks of the human body. They help build, repair, and maintain all cells, blood, and tissues in the body. Your body cannot use whole protein, but breaks it down during the process of digestion to form the type of amino acid chain it needs. All plant foods contain proteins and are the best source because they are already in the predigested, easy-to-assimilate form of amino acids. Fruits and vegetables also contain healthy fiber, vitamins, minerals, chlorophyll, antioxidants, and phytochemicals. Cooking denatures the molecular structure of protein, causing amino acids to become coagulated, and reduces the amount of usable protein. In his book *How to Get Well*, Paavo Airola notes that "you only need one half the amount the protein in your diet if you eat protein foods raw instead of cooked."

Protein from meat is highly acidic and in a form that the body cannot assimilate easily or use effectively, requiring large amounts of energy to digest. It also comes with artery-clogging cholesterol, saturated fat, hormones, and toxic residues. Excessive protein consumption can result in the accumulation of uric acid, kidney damage, over-acidity in the body, inflammation, arthritis, and a host of other health challenges. In his book *The China Study*, T. Colin Campbell states that there is a strong correlation between high amounts of dietary protein intake and cancer of the breast, prostate, pancreas, and colon.

It's easy to meet protein requirements on a raw vegan diet. Simply load up on fresh whole plant foods and remember that meat is not a necessity. It's a choice.

➤ *"The love for all living creatures is the most noble attribute of man."* —Charles Darwin

▶ *Recommended Books*

Paavo Airola: **How to Get Well; Are you Confused?; Worldwide Secrets for Staying Young;** *Mike Anderson:* **The RAVE Diet & Lifestyle; Healing Cancer from Inside Out;** *Richard Anderson:* **Cleanse & Purify Thyself;** *Neal Barnard:* **Dr. Neal Barnard's Program for Reversing Diabetes; The Cancer Survivor's Guide: Foods that Help You Fight Back; 21-Day Weight Loss Kickstart: Boost Metabolism, Lower Cholesterol, and Dramatically Improve Your Health;** *Brendan Brazier:* **Thrive Fitness: The Vegan-Based Training Program for Maximum Strength, Health, and Fitness;** *Gene Stone, editor:* **Forks Over Knives: The Plant-Based Way to Health;** *T. Colin Campbell and Thomas M. Campbell:* **The China Study: The Most Comprehensive Study of Nutrition Ever Conducted and the Startling Implications for Diet, Weight Loss and Long-Term Health;** *Brian Clement:* **Hippocrates Life Force; Living Foods for Optimum Health: Staying Healthy in an Unhealthy World; Supplements Exposed: The Truth They Don't Want You to Know About Vitamins, Minerals and Their Effects on Your Health;** *Gabriel Cousens:* **Conscious Eating; Spiritual Nutrition: Six Foundations for Spiritual Life and the Awakening of Kundalini; There is a Cure for Diabetes: The Tree of Life 21-Day+ Program;** *Joel Fuhrman:* **Eat for Health: The Mind and Body Makeover; Eat to Live: The Amazing Nutrient-Rich Program for Fast and Sustained Weight Loss; Super Immunity: The Essential Nutrition Guide for Boosting Your Body's Defenses**

to **Live Longer, Stronger, and Disease Free;** *Michael Greger:* **Bird Flu: A Virus of Our Own Hatching; Carbophobia: The Scary Truth about America's Low-Carb Craze;** *Scott Jurek:* **Eat and Run: My Unlikely Journey to Ultramarathon Greatness;** *Michael Klaper:* **Vegan Nutrition: Pure and Simple;** *John A. McDougall:* **The McDougall Program: 12 Days to Dynamic Health; The Starch Solution: Eat the Foods You Love, Regain Your Health, and Lose the Weight for Good!;** *Dean Ornish,* **Dr. Dean Ornish's Program for Reversing Heart Disease; Eat More, Weigh Less: Dr. Dean Ornish's Life Choice Program for Losing Weight Safely While Eating Abundantly;** *Rich Roll:* **Finding Ultra: Rejecting Middle Age, Becoming One of the World's Fittest Men and Discovering Myself.**

Websites of Vegan Athletes

Brendan Brazier: **brendanbrazier.com**
Scott Jurek: **scottjurek.com**
Rich Roll: **richroll.com**
Tim Van Orden: **runningraw.com**

▶ *For many years, my mother worried that my "unusual" raw diet would concern my 100-year-old Omi (meaning "grandmother" in German) in Austria. One year, when my mother, my young son, and I finally went to visit Omi, we were surprised to find that she was familiar with the raw way of eating and had even known a* **Rohköstler** *(raw foodist) who lived outside her village many years earlier.*

2. Choose Whole Foods

A healthy diet is comprised of foods found in their most natural form. These foods are whole and minimally processed, offering the highest nutrient profile for a well-balanced, healthy body. Unlike manufactured foods (which are stripped of most of their nutritional properties), whole foods are free of harmful additives, colorings, flavorings, saturated fats, sodium, and refined sugars. As an added bonus, they are high in fiber, which provides us with a sensation of fullness.

3. Eat a High Percentage of Raw Foods

Fresh raw plant foods are the centerpiece of a healthy diet. These foods offer the highest level of nutrients: everything your body needs for optimal health, vibrant energy, and life can be obtained from fresh raw vegan foods. Food is your body's fuel. If your body is clean and pure, it will thrive; but if it's overloaded with toxic pollutants, your body will degenerate and break down. Fresh fruits and vegetables should form the foundation of every meal.

Raw fruits and vegetables are the foods that are closest to nature and offer the highest level of nutrients. They are packed with valuable vitamins, minerals, enzymes, and other health-building phytochemicals. Cooking can destroy many of these nutrients, notably some water-soluble vitamins, antioxidants, heat-sensitive enzymes, and unsaturated fats, including omega-3s. Proteins and carbohydrates are rendered damaged, often producing carcinogenic compounds during the cooking process, while fiber becomes softer and less effective as an intestinal cleanser.

Whether or not you wish to go all raw, your health can benefit greatly by increasing your intake of fresh raw fruits, vegetables (especially dark leafy greens), legumes, and sprouts. Begin the day with a green smoothie or juice, followed by a bowl of fruit or chia tapioca. Try to include at least one large salad each day, and consider juicing at home so you can enjoy the benefits of raw, alkaline nutrients.

 All animals—except for humans and their domestic pets—consume their foods in a raw, uncooked state.

4. Eat Organic Foods

The toxic chemicals used on non-organic foods destroy human health and the health of our land, water, and air. Choosing organic foods is good for us *and* the environment.

Going organic means:

- keeping chemicals off our plates
- getting more nutrients from our foods
- avoiding genetically modified foods
- supporting organic farmers
- preserving ecological diversity
- protecting water quality
- eating food that tastes better
- supporting a sustainable future

If organic produce isn't available to you, you can soak produce for a few minutes in a large bowl or sink filled with water, a squeeze of lemon, and a pinch of salt, or use one of the organic vegetable and fruit washes available at most grocery stores. Alternately, peel skin of conventionally grown fruits and vegetables. The Environmental Working Group (EWG), a non-profit public interest organization dedicated to improving health and the environment, releases an annual *Dirty Dozen* list of fruits and vegetables with the highest pesticide residues. It's an excellent resource, especially if you cannot buy organics all the time. The EWG offers a downloadable pdf file, which is handy to bring when shopping, at *ewg.org*.

PLU Labels

The little sticker you often find on fruits and vegetables has a greater purpose than making the check-out process easier. Called a PLU (Price Look-Up) code, it can tell you how the produce was grown. If there are four digits and the number on the sticker begins with a 3 or a 4, the produce was conventionally grown. If there are five digits and the number on the sticker begins with a 9, the produce was grown organically. If there are five digits and the number on the sticker begins with an 8, the produce was genetically engineered (GE) or modified (GM). For example:

- *a conventionally grown apple: 4011*
- *an organic apple: 94011*
- *a GE or GM apple: 84011*

Although consumer groups and legislators have launched efforts to require labeling on genetically engineered foods, labeling remains strictly voluntary. A great way to avoid GM foods is to buy from local farmer's markets, where you can ask whether produce has been raised from GE or GM seeds.

5. Get Locally Grown Food

The nutrient content in produce begins to degrade the moment it's harvested, so unless you choose fresh produce from your local farmer's market or your own backyard, chances are that your produce was picked weeks ago, and a substantial amount of its value has been lost after picking and transport. Produce that is naturally ripened (as opposed to artificially gas ripened) is healthier and has a higher nutritional value. Many conventionally grown fruits and vegetables are harvested unripe and lack essential vitamins and minerals that naturally occur during the ripening process. To ensure that your food is as fresh as possible and that you're getting the most nutrients for your dollar, go to the farmer's market or the produce section a few times a week. Establish a relationship with your produce supplier, who may be able to provide you with special tips. I love frequenting local markets and knowing where my food is grown and, just as important, having a personal connection to the farmers who grow it.

Join a Community Supported Agriculture (CSA) network for a weekly supply of fresh local produce.

You'll get a variety of seasonal vegetables and fruits and you may even be introduced to some new ones. While it might be difficult or impossible to buy all of your food locally, any amount of food you can find and purchase locally will still benefit your health—and the planet's.

 "Tell me what you eat, and I will tell you what you are." —Jean-Anthelme Brillat-Savarin

6. Go Gluten-Free

 The word gluten comes from the Latin word meaning "glue."

Many people have recently discovered that they have difficulty digesting gluten, a glue-like protein found in various grains, including wheat, barley, spelt, kamut, and rye. Gluten is commonly found in breads and pastas, but may also be "hidden" in other foods as a filler or starch—even in salad dressings, beer, licorice, soy sauce, and many processed meat alternatives.

Symptoms of gluten intolerance can range from intestinal challenges to fatigue, joint pain, headaches, sinus congestion, bloating, and poor concentration. I have worked with many clients who have improved their health simply by eliminating gluten from their diets. I gave up eating grains in 1990, long before gluten sensitivities were acknowledged, after struggling on a grain-based, macrobiotic diet.

Gluten-free grains include quinoa, millet, buckwheat, amaranth, teff, brown rice, wild rice, and buckwheat groats. Oats are often considered gluten-free, but they may be contaminated by other grains during processing, so when purchasing oats, make sure they are certified gluten-free. If you wish to eat gluten-free grains, always soak them overnight first to remove the phytic acid and render them more digestible. There are a number of replacements for gluten-based ingredients: buckwheat, coconut, or almond flours can be used to replace grain-based flours; chia, flax seeds, and corn are alternative bases for grain-free, raw crackers; and pasta can be replaced with noodles made from fresh vegetables, including zucchini, sweet potatoes, or yams. The recipes in this book are free of ingredients that contain gluten.

The Ingredients
Fruits & Vegetables
Select fruits and vegetables from each color of the rainbow to obtain a sufficient variety of nutrients. Eat fresh fruit every day, and be sure to include apples, berries, citrus, grapes, pears, and pineapples (some of these will be available locally, depending on where you live, while some must be imported to your area). You can also buy frozen fruits or freeze your own (see note on frozen bananas, p. 43). Drying fruit is also a good way to store it; make sure your pantry includes a selection of dried apples, apricots, cranberries, figs,

goji berries, mulberries, dates, and raisins.

Leafy greens (kale, spinach, lettuce, parsley, cilantro, chard, collards, etc.) as well as sprouts (sunflower, alfalfa, broccoli, fenugreek, pea shoots, etc.) and micro-greens (baby leaves that have been grown in soil) are the staples of the whole foods raw diet. Add broccoli and cauliflower (cruciferous vegetables), avocados, bell peppers, tomatoes, carrots, zucchini, cucumbers, and fresh or dried mushrooms (shiitake mushrooms have immune-boosting properties). Sea vegetables, such as kelp, nori, dulse, and Irish moss also add nutrients and variety as well as taste to the raw diet.

> *Bananas are an excellent source of potassium, an essential mineral for our muscles, including the heart. Athletes in particular appreciate the power provided by this high-energy fruit, which makes an excellent pre-workout snack. Bananas also contain many of the B vitamins, which are necessary for proper cell formation, especially nerve cells.*
>
> *Bananas are picked off the tree while still green and unripe, but they should not be eaten until they are yellow with a few brown spots. Unripe bananas are starchy and indigestible, and eating them can cause an upset stomach.*

Fresh Herbs & Their Health Benefits

Using fresh herbs can naturally transform an ordinary meal into something extraordinary, without having to use chemical, artificial flavors. Fresh herbs add depth and fresh tastes to dishes, bring out the flavors of other ingredients, and provide balance or contrast. Herbs are not only useful in food, but also for their natural healing and health-enhancing qualities. Many drugs (such as aspirin, morphine, and tamoxifen) were originally derived from herbs.

When possible, buy organic herbs or grow your own in the garden or kitchen. Following are a few of our favorites, highlighting some of the key health benefits of each:

Basil

Aromatic and flavorful, basil also helps control blood pressure, ensures oxygen-carrying capacity in blood, and is a rich source of powerful antioxidants. Experiment with different varieties, such as sweet basil, Thai basil (which has a purple stem and mint-like flavor), and lemon basil (also popular in Thai cuisine).

Chives

Part of the onion family, but with a milder flavor, chives can be used interchangeably with recipes calling for onions. Great in raw soups, salads, garnishes, and, yes, baked potatoes, they contain antioxidants, fiber, and vitamins A, K, and B-complex.

Cilantro

Also called coriander, it has a fresh, distinct flavor that evokes strong emotions of either love or hatred in most who taste it. Often used in Mexican, Asian, and Caribbean cooking, cilantro is delicious in dressings, chutneys, chili, soups, curries, and even smoothies. It's high in vitamins A and K, and has been used to help remove toxic levels of heavy metals, such as mercury, lead, and cadmium, from the body.

Dill

A mild, aromatic herb, dill is a great way of adding extra flavor to dishes; it's excellent in soups, salads, pâtés, cheezes, and pickles. Dill can help with digestion, soothe upset stomachs, and reduce gas.

Garlic

Garlic every day keeps sickness at bay! One of the most popular and widely used flavorings throughout the world, garlic has an intense taste (and aroma), making it indispensable in any kitchen. A powerful natural antibiotic, it has been used to treat colds and flu, high blood pressure, and high cholesterol. Crushing garlic activates its therapeutic properties; crush or press it and allow it to sit for ten minutes before eating it raw.

▶ *When purchasing garlic, look for bulbs with plump, firm cloves and an intact papery outer sheath. Store bulbs in a cool dry place, but do not refrigerate.*

▶ *"In 1918, the Spanish influenza raged through Europe and claimed an estimated 20 to 50 million victims. My mother was then a teenager living in a rural area; there was no doctor nearby. When she got the flu, she was treated with raw garlic and herb teas, plum schnapps, and poultices made from raw grated potatoes." —Ilse*

Ginger

Grown in South Asia, East Africa, and the Caribbean, ginger imparts a spicy, sharp flavor to drinks, desserts, sauces, and dressings. Warming ginger is an anti-inflammatory and contains potassium, manganese, copper, and magnesium as well as vitamins B5 and B6.

▶ *Ginger is easier to grate when frozen. Peel it and store in freezer.*

Mint

Commonly grown and used around the world, mint is a refreshing addition to many dishes and adds great flavor to desserts, teas, and smoothies. It is good for digestion, reduces nausea and headaches, and soothes coughs.

Oregano

Used widely in Greek and Italian cuisine, oregano is a pungent herb with a slightly bitter taste.

It's a good source of antioxidants, vitamin C, and several important minerals.

Parsley

Whether flat-leaf or curly-leaf, parsley adds freshness and color when sprinkled over dishes as a garnish. It has natural antiseptic properties and is a good source of minerals (potassium, calcium, manganese, iron, and magnesium) and vitamins A, C, and K.

Rosemary

Common in Mediterranean and especially Italian cooking, fragrant rosemary is often added to soups, stews, salads, and teas. As an herbal remedy, rosemary is used to ease headaches. It's a source of iron, potassium, calcium, manganese, copper, and magnesium.

Sage

A pungent and slightly bitter herb, sage should be used sparingly as it can easily overpower other flavors. An antioxidant and anti-inflammatory, it's also linked with improved brain function. Sage is a rich source of minerals and is high in vitamins A and K.

Thyme

Thyme's strong fragrance and delicate flavor is good in lasagna, pâtés, dips, and dressings. Its leaves are a good source of potassium, iron, calcium, manganese, magnesium, and selenium, and of vitamins A and C.

> *Most dried herbs and spices have a shelf life of approximately six months before they begin to lose their flavor. Spices should be stored in a cool dark place, away from direct heat or light.*

Nuts & Seeds

Nuts and seeds bring a creamy consistency and rich texture to many dishes, especially desserts. Purchase raw nuts and seeds instead of roasted, and choose organic whenever possible to avoid pesticides. See below for instructions on soaking and making your own nut and seed mylks (p. 39), butters (p. 41), and flour (p. 41). Store nuts in sealed containers in the refrigerator for up to three months or in the freezer for up to one year.

Although raw nuts and seeds are nutritious and a better option than processed oils and butter, they are still high in fat and can be difficult to digest, especially when not soaked. I use very few nuts, opting instead for Irish moss or chia, flax, or hemp seeds (seeds are generally lower in fat than nuts). When I do splurge, I always balance it with plenty of high-water-content leafy greens, sprouts, and other vegetables. I also take plant-based enzymes to help with assimilation.

> *Peanuts are one of the most common food allergens. They are susceptible to aflatoxin—a mycotoxin produced by the fungus **Aspergillus flavus**, which can be highly fatal to some people.*

Chia Seeds

These little seeds are a complete protein, dense with antioxidants, omega-3 fatty acids, magnesium, zinc, iron, copper, and fiber. Unlike flax seeds, they don't require grinding to make them nutritionally accessible, nor do they become rancid. Chia seeds are available in two colors: black and white, and while there are no significant nutritional differences between them, I prefer the dark. Chia seeds have a neutral taste and can be used as a thickener in smoothies, salad dressings, sauces; dips, and desserts. They can replace eggs or other binders in recipes. For optimal bioavailability, chia seeds should be soaked for at least four hours before using.

The dry whole seeds can be stored at room temperature. Gluten-free chia seeds make a satisfying breakfast and can be topped with mylk and fresh fruit. They're high in essential fatty acids, calcium, antioxidants, and iron. Chia seeds are also an excellent source of dietary fiber and provide natural long-lasting energy to keep you running like the Aztecs!

Coconut Oil & Butter

Coconut oil is high in lauric acid, which has antiviral, antimicrobial, and antifungal properties. It is used to make sauces, desserts, and smoothies—and also makes a great face and body cream. Coconut butter includes both the oil and flesh of coconuts. It is a naturally sweet, rich and creamy spread that can also complement desserts, soups, and smoothies. Coconut oil has a melting point of about 76°F (24°C); below that temperature, the oil will solidify.

Many recipes in this book call for melted coconut oil. To melt, submerge a sealed glass jar of coconut oil in a deep bowl of hot water for about 5–10 minutes. Alternatively, place a jar of coconut oil on top of running dehydrator or warm oven until it melts.

Sweeteners

There's no reason to use white sugar when there are so many healthier (and tastier) alternatives, most of which are not very expensive. If you care about your health, avoid all foods that contain high-fructose corn syrup. Healthier alternatives include:

Coconut palm sugar or coconut nectar are not raw, but are low-glycemic, delicious, and nutritious alternatives to processed cane sugar.

Dates and date paste (see p. 43) are rich in antioxidants and are among the most alkaline of foods. They are a great source of potassium, iron, vitamin A, magnesium, selenium, and fiber. There are many varieties of dates, but I like Medjool best (known as the "king of dates"); they are exceptionally plump, sweet, and have a delicious, rich caramel-like taste. Whole dates can be stored for up to six months in the refrigerator.

Honey is a byproduct of bees, so many vegans choose not to eat it.

Lucuma powder, derived from a Peruvian fruit, is often used as a low-glycemic sweetener in the raw world; it has a subtle caramel flavor.

Maple syrup or maple sugar are not raw, but are high in minerals. I buy organic maple syrup from a local farmer.

Stevia is an herb that has been used for centuries as a sweetener in South America. The extract from the stevia leaf is very sweet, with 300 times the sweetness of sugar, yet it's calorie-free. It doesn't raise blood-sugar levels and so is safe for people with diabetes. Stevia is available as a powder or liquid (the green powder is less processed).

The healthiest sweetener is **whole, soaked fruits** (dates, raisins, apricots, figs).

 A note on agave

*When I wrote **The SimplyRaw Living Foods Detox Manual** in 2008, raw agave had just hit the market. It was touted as "the" great raw low-glycemic sweetener. Like many others, I hopped on the agave bandwagon, replacing maple syrup with agave. Recently, however, agave has become controversial because it is highly processed and has a high fructose content. I have since returned to using maple syrup and stevia as my sweeteners of choice.*

The Tools

While having the right kitchen tools certainly makes food preparation easier, it is not a prerequisite to eating healthily. When I first transitioned to a raw diet, I had very few kitchen appliances other than a low-end juicer, an inexpensive knife, and a wooden salad bowl, but I still managed to prepare wholesome and pleasing meals. I ate predominately whole fruits, simple salad combinations, fresh vegetable juices, and sprouts, along with some soaked nuts, seeds, wheatgrass, and algae. These foods form the foundation of the living foods lifestyle developed by Dr Ann Wigmore, from which many raw foodists, unfortunately, have since strayed.

My kitchen is now outfitted with time-saving tools that help me to prepare a wide variety of raw meals. These tools also come in handy for my food-prep classes as well as spontaneous, in-the-moment creations. While I have two dehydrators at home (we don't own an oven), I rarely turn them on except in workshops or occasionally during the colder months when I'm in need of denser (i.e., more concentrated and filling) foods.

Many recipes in this book can be prepared with no more than a decent cutting knife, a grater, or standard blender—in other words, you don't have to wait until you have the perfect equipment set-up in order to transition to raw foods. Most kitchens already have what's required; work with what you have, and gradually add to your collection of kitchen tools. You can chop by hand if you don't have a food processor or mandoline; use a vegetable peeler instead of a spiralizer for noodles; and if a recipe calls for dehydration and you don't have a dehydrator, simply turn the oven on to its lowest temperature and leave the door slightly ajar. If you're craving fresh juice but don't have a juicer, blend vegetables with a few cups of water in a blender, then strain the juice through a cheesecloth or nut mylk bag. And if you don't have a nut mylk bag, use a piece of pantyhose (clean, of course!) instead—it really works!

When you are ready to add more kitchen tools, you don't have to buy everything new. Explore second-hand stores, garage sales, and online sources in your area. I've discovered many gems while rummaging through other people's discards—including a Champion juicer, a few decent food processors, a dehydrator, and even an old, but new to me, Vitamix stainless steel blender.

I find the following tools useful when preparing whole raw foods:

- **Bamboo mat**: For sushi makers. With some practice, you can roll sushi without one, but it helps to maintain even pressure on the sushi roll, giving an even finish.
- **Cheesecloth**: A gauze-like cotton used primarily for making nut cheeze.

- **Citrus zester**: Lemon or orange zest adds color and flair to many recipes.
- **Cutting board**: Wood, bamboo, or plastic—a must-have.
- **Garlic press**: Crushes ginger, too.
- **Grater/shredder**: My mother and I would be lost in the kitchen without our graters, which are useful for creating different textures from vegetables. Grating also makes vegetables easier to digest.
- **Hand citrus juicer**: Less expensive (and, in my opinion, less messy) than an electric juicer, the one I use is wooden and costs only a few dollars.
- **Knives in different sizes**: A sharp knife is the chef's best friend. Ceramic knives are lightweight and remain sharp forever; they make cutting ultra easy and help prevent oxidation of food.
- **Mandoline**: The razor-sharp blade slices vegetables into uniform, paper-thin slices for lasagna noodles, wrappers, cannelloni, etc.
- **Mason (canning) jars**: These indispensable glass containers with screw-top lids are used to soak, sprout, and store food.
- **Measuring cups and spoons**: How else will you know the difference between a teaspoon and a tablespoon?

- **Nut mylk bag**: Important for making smooth, homemade non-dairy mylks, it is also handy for making nut cheezes.
- **Potato peeler**: Shred veggies into thin even strips or make vegetable noodles.
- **Rubber spatulas**: For spreading, scraping, and licking—you can't have enough of them!
- **Salad bowl**: Treat yourself to a wooden or bamboo salad bowl for mixing and serving your delicious creations.
- **Salad spinner**: Useful for drying leafy veggies, and it makes a big difference in keeping your salads crispy.
- **Silicone molds**: For making chocolates and other desserts.
- **Spiral slicer**: By far the best little hand-operated gadget invented, it's also fairly inexpensive and can transform zucchini, beets, yams, turnips, and other hard vegetables into fabulous "noodles."
- **Springform pans** (sometimes called flan pans): These have removable bottoms and come in various shapes and sizes.
- **Squeeze bottles**: Inexpensive and great for drizzling sauces and dressings.
- **Steamer**: An inexpensive basket-shaped steamer that sits inside a pot is vital for lightly cooking vegetables.

- **Strainer/colander**: Rinse fruit and veg, soaked nuts, and fermented nut cheeze.

Electrical appliances

In addition to the hand tools listed above, the following electrical appliances can save time and effort:

- **Blender**: Create creamy smoothies, nut mylks, dressings, sauces, cheezes, soups, desserts, and juice. A high-speed blender, such as a Vitamix or Blendtec, works best, but any blender will do; just blend a little longer with a lower-powered one.
- **Coffee grinder**: Use it to grind salt, spices, and small amounts of nuts or seeds.
- **Dehydrator**: It may not be essential for living the raw life, but it does make it more interesting, as a dehydrator allows you to "bake" (at a low temperature that doesn't destroy enzymes) raw crackers, breads, granola, fruit leathers, trail mixes, crusts, and, of course, your very own kale chips.
- **Food processor**: Useful for making pâtés, nut butters, pie crusts, brownies, and soups and sauces with a chunky texture.
- **Juicer**: Juices will take your health to new heights. When shopping for a juicer, you may wish to find one that processes not only fruits and vegetables, but also wheatgrass.

- **Rice cooker:** Not for the raw foodist, but if you have to cook for a family, it's useful for cooking all kinds of grains and prevents them from burning. We purchased one recently to cook quinoa for my teenage son.

 My mother likes to cook in a cast-iron pan, as the iron is absorbed into the food.

The Techniques

Raw cuisine is different from traditional cooking in many ways, and to a novice it can appear complicated, foreign, and time-consuming. Although there is an initial learning curve, preparing raw meals can be quite simple—often simpler than cooking. The following basic techniques form the foundation for making a variety of raw food recipes.

 Avoid cooking with oil

The omega-3s in vegetable oils are unstable and easily oxidized by heat. Cooking can cause the fats to release free radicals; when consumed, free radicals can damage cells, leading to inflammation and contributing to heart disease. Consuming cooked oils can also lead to skin issues including eczema and clogged pores.

For cooked meals, use water instead of oil to "sauté" foods in a pan. Use a good quality stainless steel or cast iron frying pan, and stir frequently. Another great alternative to cooking foods in oil is to lightly steam them; nutrients are better retained when foods are steamed than when they're boiled or fried.

Making Vegetable "Pastas"

Spiralized noodles made from zucchini, carrots, beets, parsnips, sweet potatoes, turnips, jicama, cucumbers, daikon, rutabaga, parsnips, and squash are so much tastier than cooked, processed pastas. Not only are vegetable noodles light and low in carbohydrates, they are amazingly delicious. Even fussy eaters will enjoy eating vegetables when they've been transformed into something delicate and visually appealing, especially when tossed with a flavorful sauce. Preparing veggie noodles with children is a fun way of involving them in meal-making.

My favorite noodles are made from zucchinis; they're neutral in flavor, high in water content, and easy to digest. It only takes a few minutes to make a bowl of zucchini noodles, especially if you have a spiral slicer. You can peel off the skins or leave them on for the dark green color and extra nutrition they provide. Zucchini peels can sometimes be bitter, so taste before peeling.

If you don't have a spiral slicer or spiralizer, use a potato peeler, mandoline, or julienne peeler. I often use a potato peeler; it may take a little bit longer to make noodles, but the clean-up is faster than if using a spiralizer. Here are a few ways of making noodles using some of the tools mentioned above:

- **Julienne peeler**: An inexpensive julienne peeler is great alternative to a spiral slicer. Although it can be somewhat tricky to peel close to the bottom of the zucchini, the peeler creates thin noodles as well as a spiralizer, and you won't have a machine to clean.
- **Mandoline**: A mandoline makes long thin julienne strips from an uncut, full-length zucchini. The blades are very sharp—use caution!
- **Potato peeler**: Peel zucchini lengthwise into 1/8–1/4-in (3–6-mm) thick strips. Don't use the inside section that contains the seeds. Cut strips lengthwise into long thin "noodles."
- **Spiral slicer (spiralizer)**: Make sure the zucchinis are firm and fairly straight. The wider the zucchini, the bigger (and better) the noodle. Cut off ends, and if the zucchini is long, slice into 2 or 3 lengths. Select the blade setting and start spiralizing your zucchini into thin, pasta-like strands.

Soaking Nuts & Seeds

Nuts and seeds are little powerhouses, offering a wealth of healthy fats, amino acids (protein), fiber, vitamins, minerals, and enzymes essential for optimal health. They are a wonderful addition to every diet.

However, nuts and seeds contain metabolic inhibitors that protect them from bacterial invasion and keep them dormant. Phytic acid, for instance, binds to important minerals (particularly calcium, iron, zinc, and magnesium) in the gastrointestinal tract, and can interfere with their absorption and result in mineral deficiencies. Soaking nuts and seeds in purified water removes the phytic acid, releases enzymes, and starts the germination process. (In nature, enzyme inhibitors and other compounds are removed once the proper conditions for growth—rain, soil, and sunlight—are met. When damp, the seed germinates and begins to sprout and produce a plant. The plant continues to grow in sunlight.) During the germination process, the nutritional value and digestibility of the seed are improved. Enzyme inhibitors, phytates (natural insecticides), and oxalates (which shield the seed from oxygen) are removed, and "pre-digestion" occurs: starches are broken down into simple sugars; proteins are converted into amino acids; and fats are broken down into soluble fatty acids. The fat or oil content is slightly reduced after soaking, too, as some of it is released into the water.

Many cultures around the world have known about the value of soaking (and fermenting) nuts, seeds, legumes, and grains before consuming them. The ancient Aztecs, for instance, soaked seeds overnight before drying them in the sunlight. Indians ferment rice and lentils to make dosas, a fermented crêpe or pancake, and the Japanese ferment soy beans to produce miso and soy sauce. Raw foodists are rediscovering the nutritional value of soaking nuts and seeds.

➤ *Ideally, grains and legumes should also be soaked overnight (6–12 hours) prior to cooking. This neutralizes enzyme inhibitors and phytates, making grains more digestible and nutrients more bioavailable. Soaking also reduces cooking time. To soak grains, place in a bowl with double the amount of purified water. Rinse before cooking.*

I find that my body can digest nuts and seeds much easier when they've been soaked, and even easier, when fermented. As a raw foodist, I believe that eating a diet heavy in un-soaked nuts and seeds can be less healthy than one in which some lightly cooked, whole plant foods are eaten. To put things into perspective, un-soaked nuts and seeds are better than foods made with processed flours, butter, white sugar, or hydrogenated oils. (There is always a "better than" option to choose!) I recommend digestive enzymes if you eat nuts without soaking them; enzymes can help the body break down and absorb the nuts more easily.

Raw recipes which depend on a crumbly texture call for "dry" nuts and seeds. Soak nuts first, then dehydrate them for 12–16 hours, or until dry, in a dehydrator or at the lowest temperature in an oven with the door ajar. If you don't have a dehydrator or are in a rush, just use raw unsoaked nuts and seeds. Although not ideal, small amounts of unsoaked nuts and seeds are better than oil roasted. Chew them

thoroughly to aid digestion. Soaked nuts and seeds are best; raw and unsoaked are second best.

➤ ***Timesaving tip***: *Soak and dehydrate batches of nuts and seeds in advance and store in glass jars to have them readily available for recipes.*

Soaking times vary with the size of the nut or seed; the smaller they are, the less soaking time is required. Although there are many complicated soaking charts available, the most important thing to remember is to just soak nuts and seeds before eating them. I generally soak them in the evenings before going to bed, then drain and rinse them in the morning, and store them in the refrigerator. Light colored nuts—like cashews, macadamia, and pine nuts—do not need to be soaked, but soaking for 30 minutes makes blending smoother, especially important for cheeze, dessert, and sauce recipes. Hemp seeds don't need to be soaked at all, as they are very small and tender.

➤ *To soak nuts and seeds:*
  - *Place nuts or seeds in a colander and rinse well.*
  - *Transfer to a wide-mouthed canning jar or glass bowl.*
  - *Cover one part nuts or seeds with two parts purified water; for instance, 1 cup (250 mL) almonds to 2 cups (500 mL) water.*
  - *Cover with breathable dish cloth or cheesecloth. Place on counter or in refrigerator and soak overnight or between four and eighteen hours.*

- *Rinse well and discard soak water, which contains enzyme inhibitors.*
- *Store soaked and air dried (or dehydrated) nuts or seeds in an airtight container in the refrigerator. Soaked nuts and seeds will last for up to five days.*

Some soaked seeds will begin to sprout, which is a great way to make them more alkaline and increase their nutrient profile. Sprouted seeds make an excellent addition to salads, smoothies, sandwiches, soups, and garnishes.

Chia seeds absorb up to 10 times their own weight in water. Once soaked, the seeds swell and become gelatinous, which makes them very filling.

▶ *To soak chia seeds:*

⅓ cup (80 mL) chia seeds
2 cups (500 mL) water

Add chia seeds and water to a small bowl. Stir well to prevent clumping. Let soak for at least 4 hours. Store in a sealed container for up to 10 days in the refrigerator.
Makes about 2 cups.

Soaking Buckwheat

Buckwheat is versatile and popular among raw foodists, especially during the winter months as it has a warming effect on the body. (**Note:** Purchase raw hulled buckwheat groats.) Soaked buckwheat can be used in cereals, porridge, sprinkled over salads, and dehydrated into crunchy "buckwheaties" to nibble on as a snack. Sprouting buckwheat is very simple: Soak 1 part buckwheat in 2 parts water for 15 minutes. (It will develop a starchy, slimy coating if soaked for longer.) Rinse well before draining, and leave it in a colander (covered with a cloth) overnight (8–16 hours). Rinse again before using.

Homemade Nut & Seed Mylks

Nuts and seeds make delicious milk alternatives or "mylks," naturally packed with vitamins, minerals, protein, beneficial enzymes, and antioxidants. They are a much healthier alternative to cow's milk and provide us with the familiar taste and texture found in dairy, but without the unhealthy animal fats and antibiotics and hormones found in conventional (i.e., not organic) dairy milk (see "The Scoop on Dairy," p. 40).

Although it's easy to find milk alternatives at most grocery stores, manufactured "health foods" can contain fillers, processed sweeteners, and additives that are not optimal for our health. While boxed mylks are an improvement over animal milk, you can make your own nutritious and creamy mylks economically and with very little effort. Homemade milk alternatives are fresh, nourishing, enzyme-rich, and free from processed sugars, preservatives, or other harmful ingredients. They have a surprisingly rich, delicious flavor, and you won't be wasting milk cartons or contributing packaging to landfills. Nut and seed mylks can be used in smoothies to replace milk or yogurt, poured over cereals, added to your morning brew, or simply enjoyed on their own.

You can make any kind of mylk you want, using organic almonds, pecans, cashews, hazelnuts, macadamias, coconuts, or Brazil nuts, or pumpkin, sunflower, sesame, or hemp seeds. Customize the flavor and sweetness, or leave it plain and unsweetened. Vary the types of nuts or seeds you choose to obtain a wide variety of nutrients, and experiment with different sweeteners, including dates, apricots, coconut sugar, maple syrup, stevia, lucuma, or raw honey, and various spices such as vanilla, cinnamon, cardamom, or nutmeg. You'll be surprised at all the delicious possibilities! See the basic nut or seed mylk recipe on p. 60.

Nut and seed pulp can be dehydrated (or baked at a low temperature) for 8–12 hours and used in pie crusts, granola, bread, cookies, cakes, or cracker recipes, or simply add it to fresh or dried fruit and top with mylk. It also freezes well. Leftover almond pulp makes a good natural facial scrub.

> *Nut mylk bags are easier to clean when used inside out, as most bags have a seam where pulp can accumulate. To clean nut mylk bag, scrub with natural dish soap, soak in a bowl of water, and rinse thoroughly. Hang to air dry over your sink.*

> *Brazil nuts contain exceptionally high levels of selenium, a powerful trace mineral and important co-factor for the enzyme glutathione peroxidase. Selenium helps protect the body from free-radical damage and gives it ammunition to fight diseases. Selenium deficiencies occur in areas where soils are poor.*

The Scoop on Dairy

"Cow's milk in the past has always been oversold as the perfect food, but we are now seeing that it isn't the perfect food at all and the government really shouldn't be behind any efforts to promote it as such." —**Benjamin Spock**

Many of us were raised to believe that cow's milk was the perfect food. The dairy industry spends millions of dollars every year on advertising campaigns to brainwash the public into thinking that "milk does the body good." Nothing could be further from the truth.

Milk is touted as a major source of calcium. (How often have we heard from the dairy industry that if we don't drink milk, our bones will become brittle and our teeth will fall out?) However, most leafy greens, fruits, vegetables, nuts, and seeds are also excellent sources of calcium. Milk and other dairy products create an acidic environment in the body, which leads to the leaching of calcium from bones.

According to *The China Study*, "Dairy intake is one of the most consistent dietary predictors for prostate cancer in the published literature, and those who consume the most dairy have double to quadruple the risk." Milk contains saturated fats, growth hormones, allergens, and the protein casein, which has been linked to cancer. Milk consumption has been linked to heart disease, obesity, diabetes, asthma, eczema, constipation, gas, irritable bowel syndrome, sinus congestion, diminished immunity, earaches, and allergies. It also creates excess mucus in the body.

Adults do not need to drink milk of any kind. Infants need milk—their mother's milk. Cow's milk is meant to nourish baby cows and help them grow from their birth weight of about seventy pounds (thirty-two kg) to about 1,000 pounds (454 kg) in their first year. Human beings do not need the milk that baby cows do. Humans are the only species on the planet that choose to drink the milk of another animal. Just as dog's milk is intended for puppies, cat's milk for kittens, and human's milk for human infants, cow's milk is meant for calves.

> *"When I was eight years old, I went with my mother to get milk from the local farmer. On the way home, we greeted an elderly man who was busy placing sliced fruit and vegetables on a white sheet spread over the grass to dry in the sun. When he saw the milk canister my mother was carrying, he said, 'Why do you let your little girl drink milk? It is harmful to your gut!' Later, my mother explained to me that he was a* **Rohköstler**, *a raw foodist." —Ilse*

Making Nut & Seed Butters

Organic raw nut butters can be expensive, but making your own is easy and economical, though it requires a little patience. Homemade raw nut and seed butters are as flavorful as store-bought, but without the excess salt, sugar, oil, and other hidden ingredients, and you can customize the flavor and texture to suit your tastes (see p. 142).

Process nuts or seeds in a food processor. You may have to turn it off periodically to avoid overheating it. Scrape nut butter from the sides with a spatula before turning it on again. Continue processing until desired texture is reached. It can take about 15 minutes to get a creamy nut butter. (To make your own coconut butter, see p. 145.)

Making Nut & Seed Flour

Freshly ground nuts and seeds give desserts a delicate texture and flavor. Nut flours are also a great way to use up nut pulp (after it's been dried) left over from making nut mylk.

Easy Homemade Almond Flour

- 3 cups (750 mL) raw almonds
- In blender or food processor, add almonds 1 cup (250 mL) at a time and grind to a fine powder, about 30 seconds.
- Makes approximately 2½ cups (625 mL).

▶ *All almonds originating from the US are pasteurized. I use Sicilian or Spanish raw almonds, which are unpasteurized.*

Ground shredded coconut makes a delicious, light gluten- and nut-free flour alternative:

Simple Coconut Flour

- 4 cups (1 L) shredded coconut
- Blend coconut in a blender or food processor to create a delicious gluten-free flour.
- Makes approximately 3 cups (750 mL).

▶ *Flax seeds are an outstanding food, rich in fiber, lignans, and omega-3 fatty acids. However, whole flax seeds are not easy to digest and need to be ground into a powder.*
    To make your own flax meal, simply grind whole flax seeds (I prefer the mild taste of golden flax) in a coffee grinder. Once ground, they go rancid quickly, so use them immediately or store briefly in the refrigerator.

Ripening Fruit

Much fruit is picked unripe and shipped to market when it's not at its nutritional peak. Eating unripe fruit can cause digestive upset (bloating, gas, constipation). If you want to accelerate the ripening process, place fruit in a dry paper bag. Close it and store out of direct sunlight at room temperature. To further speed up the process, place a banana inside the bag with the other fruit; bananas give off ethylene, a natural gas that will hasten ripening. Check fruit each day; once ripe, store in the refrigerator. (**Note:** Never refrigerate bananas and tomatoes; they'll lose flavor!)

Dried Fruit

Dried fruits such as dates, raisins, figs, goji berries, prunes, apricots, mangos, pineapples, and cranberries are some of the healthiest alternatives to sugar, and a great way to satisfy a sweet craving. They are an excellent solution for the traveler, as good nourishment is not always available on the road. Dried fruits can be soaked to soften and render them more digestible before using in recipes. Place them in a bowl, cover with water, and let sit for at least 30 minutes before adding to smoothies and desserts or sprinkling over a salad. Save the soak water and use as a liquid sweetener.

Drying food is one of the oldest methods of preserving fruit and vegetables. It is a simple and cost-efficient way to use ripe produce at peak season when favorite local fruits, vegetables, and herbs are abundant and inexpensive. Dried fruits make the perfect healthy treat for children; they are lightweight and can be easily packed for nutritious snacks, lunches, and hiking trips.

If you don't have a dehydrator, use your oven at a low temperature (below 200°F/95°C) and be sure to leave the oven door ajar to maintain air circulation during the drying process. Once moisture has been removed from the food, you can store it in glass jars for long periods without refrigeration.

> ➤ *Always purchase organic dried fruits, as conventional ones contain sulfites, chemical compounds used to increase their shelf life and retain their color. Sulfites can cause headaches, breathing difficulties, and other allergic reactions. Packaged dried fruits may also contain added sugar, so always remember to check the ingredient list.*

Date paste is an excellent natural sweetener full of valuable nutrients and fiber (which helps slow down blood-sugar spikes); it's a healthy alternative to other sweeteners. This is a basic recipe for date paste, which can be used to add a touch of sweetness to smoothies, salad dressings, sauces, desserts, and more.

Date Paste

- 1 cup (250 mL) pitted dates
- a squeeze of lemon juice (to help preserve freshness)
- In a bowl, cover dates with cold water and soak for one hour. Remove dates and reserve water. In a food processor, purée dates with lemon juice until thick and creamy. Adjust

consistency with the reserved soak water, if needed. If you don't have a blender or food processor, simply mash pitted dates by hand or with a mortar and pestle without water.
- Makes about 1 cup (250 mL).

Transfer to an airtight container and store in refrigerator. Date paste will keep approximately two to three weeks in the refrigerator, or up to three months in the freezer. (**Tip:** Label the container so you remember when you made it. If freezing date paste, store it in a resealable freezer bag or plastic container so you can break off pieces as you need them.)

> ➤ *My Moldovan father went to school in Istanbul where dates were a staple food. They continued to be a family tradition in Canada where we ate them regularly instead of chocolate and other sugary sweets. Full of minerals, dates are a great way to give yourself a natural energy boost during the day.*

Freezing Bananas

Freezing is a great way to save over-ripe bananas. I frequently load up on spotted, price-reduced, organic bananas and take them home to freeze. Frozen bananas give a cold and sweet creaminess to smoothies, transforming a mediocre smoothie into something special. Use in place of ice cubes, which water down the flavor. Frozen bananas can also be used in puddings, ice creams, banana bread, muffins, or pancakes.

To freeze, simply peel the banana, cut it into slices, and put them in a freezer bag. Seal and date the bag. Frozen bananas should be used within two to three months.

Preparing Irish Moss

Irish moss is a red seaweed rich in nutrients, particularly minerals and antioxidants. It has a soothing effect on the stomach and is said to ease indigestion, nausea, and ulcers. Irish moss has also been used to help treat bronchitis and can soothe skin conditions such as eczema, psoriasis, and burns when applied topically. The carrageenan extracted from Irish moss is used as a thickening agent in many foods and cosmetics.

Recently, Irish moss has become popular among raw foodists for its natural thickening properties. It is the raw vegan answer to gelatin! I often use it to reduce my nut intake in desserts without compromising the creamy texture. It also enhances dressings, sauces, pie fillings, and cakes, making them lighter and fluffier.

To prepare Irish moss:

1. Place about 1 cup (250 mL) Irish moss in a colander or sieve.
2. Rinse well under cold running water to remove all sand and grit. Rinse and repeat a few times until clean.
3. Place in bowl or a Mason jar and cover completely with purified water.
4. Set in the refrigerator and allow to soak for eight to twelve hours.
5. Remove from refrigerator and rinse again with cold water.
6. Place Irish moss in blender, adding three-quarters the amount of purified water to cover.
7. Blend until smooth, adding more water 1 tbsp at a time as needed to achieve a thick, smooth paste.
8. Use right away or transfer to a clean canning jar and store in refrigerator for up to three weeks.

 Always use cold water when preparing Irish moss. Using warm or hot water will cause it to release its gelling properties into the water.

Making Celery Powder

If you're on a low-sodium diet, use celery powder (not celery salt) as the optimal salt alternative. It's easy to make your own:

- 1 bunch celery
- Chop celery into thin slices. Spread slices on dehydrator trays and dehydrate (105°F [41°C]) for about 12 hours or until dry. (Or place slices on baking sheets and dry in oven on lowest temperature with door slightly ajar until dry.) In a blender or food processor, grind dried celery until it forms a fine powder. Store in an airtight container.

Warming Raw Foods

Most foods are best when eaten at room temperature rather than cold. Many people want to eat heated foods during the colder months of the year. This craving for warmth can present a dilemma for raw foodists and those transitioning to raw, but there are some simple ways to warm foods gently without destroying their enzyme content:

- Remove foods from refrigerator one-half to one hour before eating.
- Place food in dehydrator at 105°F (41°C) or in oven on the lowest temperature with the door slightly ajar for thirty minutes, until warmed.
- Lightly warm food on stove top until warm to the touch.
- Add spices to provide some internal warmth.
- Heat bowl or dish before plating food.
- Wash refrigerated produce in warm water or set in a bowl of warm water for a few moments before using.
- Warm soups and sauces by blending in a high-speed blender or food processor for a few minutes.
- Use warm water in soups.

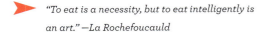 *"To eat is a necessity, but to eat intelligently is an art." —La Rochefoucauld*

Balancing Flavors

"Season to taste." Three simple words that can make all the difference between a bland dish and one that bursts with flavor. Season to taste means letting your own taste buds guide you; there is no right or wrong. The most important thing to remember is to add a small amount of seasoning at a time, and taste as you go along. There are a few basic flavors that, when combined, truly enhance a dish. Balance these flavors to give your meals depth:

Sweet

fresh and dried fruits, maple syrup, stevia, lucuma, carob, tomatoes, red bell peppers, cashews

Salty

Himalayan salt, miso, tamari, sun-dried tomatoes, olives, dulse and other sea vegetables

Sour

lemons, limes, oranges, grapefruits, cranberries, vinegar, sauerkraut, tamarind

Bitter

dandelion greens, arugula, romaine, kale, parsley, basil, nutmeg, cumin

Savory

sage, oregano, basil, cumin, cinnamon

Spicy/pungent

ginger, garlic, onions, cayenne pepper and other hot chili peppers, mustard

Note: fats or oils (avocados, nuts, seeds) can help carry the flavors and bring all the elements together!

If you find that a dish seems to be "missing something," it may be out of balance:

- Too spicy/pungent? Balance with sweet or fat
- Too sweet? Balance with sour, fat, or salt
- Too sour? Balance with sweet, salt, fat, or bitter
- Too salty? Balance with sweet, sour, or fat
- Too bland? Add sweet, sour, and a touch of sour or spicy
- Needs more depth? Add savory

The following recipes are 100-percent gluten-free and 100-percent plant-based, and most of them are raw. Over many years, I have tested and adapted them at SimplyRaw workshops, classes, and events. I've served most of them to my family and to customers at my mainly raw restaurant in Ottawa, Canada, SimplyRaw Express, so they have been taste-tested by thousands of people—mostly mainstream non-vegetarians.

While I know that these recipes will delight your families and friends, I encourage you to be creative with them—experiment with and adjust them to your own tastes. There are countless delicious variations! Be imaginative, taste as you go, have fun, and play with the flavors as you make these recipes your own.

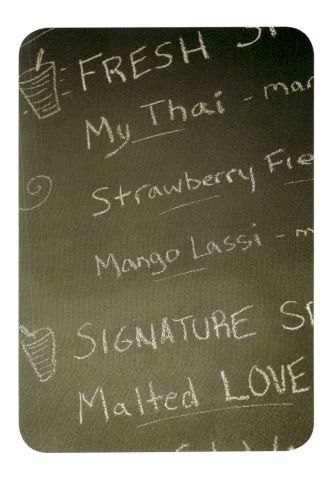

Key to symbols

 = Cooked foods

 = Contains nuts

 = An ingredient must be soaked for 30 minutes or more. In some recipes, soaking and then dehydrating nuts and seeds is the best option, but it is optional; raw, dry nuts can be used instead.

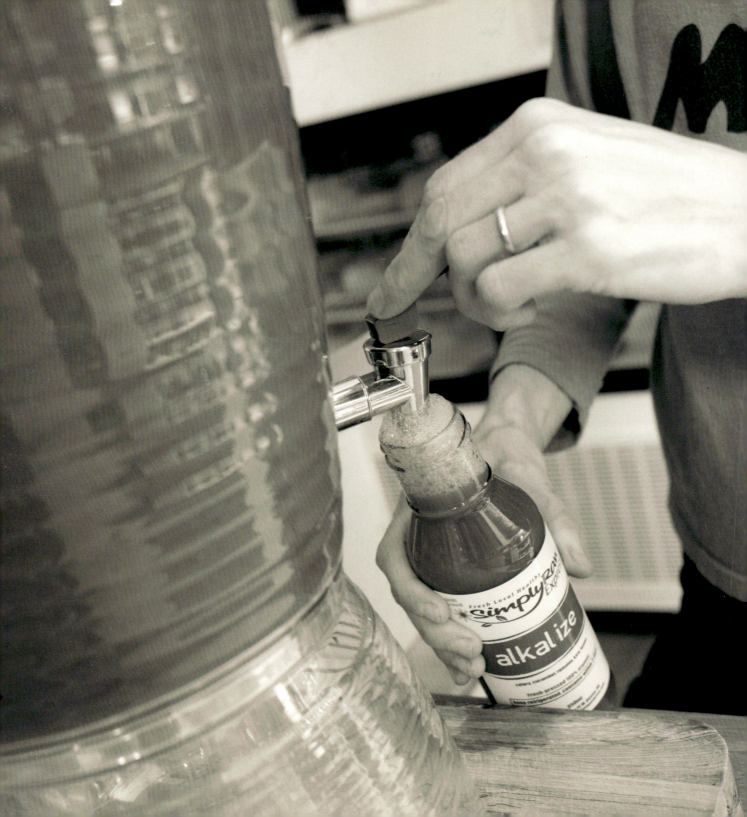

BEVERAGES

My Daily Greens   51

Liquid Gold   52

Kick Acid   52

Inflammation Buster   53

Watermelon Cooler   54

Anti-Ulcer Cocktail   55

Sweet Green Monster   56

My Thai Smoothie   56

Strawberry Fields Smoothie 57

Tropical Mint Smoothie   58

Mango Lassi   58

Shamrock Mint Chip Shake 59

Choc-O-Love Shake   60

Basic Nut or Seed Mylk   60

Sugar-Kissed Pecan Mylk 61

One-Minute Miracle Mylk 61

Vanilla Almond Mylk   62

Instant Hemp Mylk   64

Do-It-Yourself Coconut Mylk 64

About Thai Coconuts   65

Vanilla Bean Bubble Mylk 66

Yogi Tea   67

Sun Tea   68

Holiday Nut Nog   68

Warmed White Chocolate   69

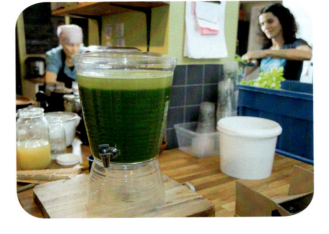

Leafy greens and other vegetables are nutritional superstars—powerful sources of health- and immune-building vitamins, minerals, enzymes, antioxidants, and other important nutrients that keep you vibrant, energized, and nourished. Vegetable juices are alkaline, and consuming enough of them will help to ensure that the body doesn't become overly acidic, which some nutritionists believe is at the root of many diseases and conditions.

Eating fiber-rich plant foods uncooked preserves their essential nutrients, but the high-fiber content can be difficult to digest. Blending and juicing allow us to increase our fruit and vegetable intake—in larger quantities than if we were to consume them whole—in easy-to-digest liquid forms, making the nutrients more readily available to the body. Juices and smoothies, however, serve two different yet equally important roles. Juicing extracts the nutrients and filters out the fiber, so the body does not have to work as hard to break down the food. Smoothies contain all of the fiber from the fruits and vegetables, but the blending process helps to break down the fiber and makes it easier to digest. Smoothies are more filling and quicker to prepare than juices; they make fast, convenient meals.

There is debate over which—juices or smoothies—is better, but both green juices and smoothies are important elements in my diet. While I am very loyal to my juicer and generally drink one quart/liter of fresh juice daily, I also make and enjoy my share of green smoothies. I recommend varying the fruits and veggies you drink or eat; different foods offer different nutrients. Juices and smoothies are great for using up leftover vegetables in the refrigerator, so if you don't have some of the ingredients in the recipes that follow, feel free to be creative, and juice what you have on hand.

Fresh juice is quite delicate. Once exposed to oxygen, the precious nutrients begin to degrade. To minimize this oxidation, it is always best to consume immediately following extraction. If you cannot drink it right away, pour the juice into a bottle, ensuring that it is filled right to the top with little air space, and store in the refrigerator.

➤ *While I recommend that you invest in a good quality blender and juicer, these tools are not critical for a raw diet. Better quality machines do have an effect on the quality of the drinks—both nutritionally and for texture and consistency—but even a simple blender or juicer are better than nothing. (Look for a used machine; someone else's rubbish could be your gold!)*

MY DAILY GREENS

MAKES ABOUT 1 QT/L

I often make this juice while working from home. It is my all-time favorite liquid lunch that keeps me going for hours. Add a clove or 2 of garlic during flu season. If you can't tolerate fruit sugar, omit the apple and add some lemon juice.

1 head romaine lettuce

3 cups (750 mL) mixed sprouts (sunflower, pea shoots, alfalfa and/or fenugreek)

6 celery stalks

5 kale leaves and stalks

3 Jerusalem artichokes

2 tsp chopped fresh ginger

2 whole apples, quartered and cored

2–3 garlic cloves (optional)

In a juicer, process all ingredients and drink right away.

▶ *Often called sunchokes, Jerusalem artichokes resemble gnarly little potatoes. They are not related to artichokes but to sunflowers! High in the prebiotic inulin, which stimulates the growth of bifidobacteria in the intestines, they are a good source of potassium (more than found in bananas), protein, and vitamin C.*

▶ *I add Jerusalem artichokes to most of my juices. Make sure to clean them with a vegetable scrubber before consuming.*

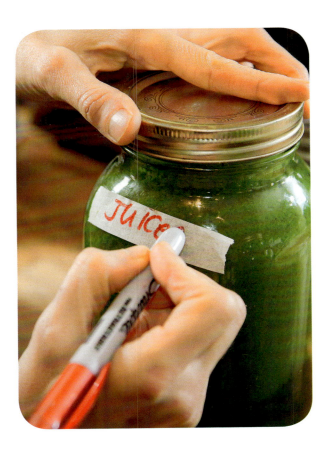

LIQUID GOLD

MAKES 1 SERVING

If you're looking for the elixir of life, look no further. Grab some wheatgrass, and get ready for some serious business! Drink Liquid Gold on an empty stomach, as wheatgrass juice can cause nausea when consumed soon after meals. Wait at least an hour before eating or drinking. Wheatgrass juice should be consumed within 10 minutes of juicing so its nutrients don't begin to diminish.

> *Because of its high chlorophyll content, wheatgrass juice is a powerful detoxifier and blood builder. Popularized by Dr Ann Wigmore, it has been used to boost the immune system and oxygenate the cells. Wheatgrass is also abundant in vitamins A, B, C, and E, as well as oxygen, amino acids (protein), enzymes, and minerals.*

3–4 handfuls wheatgrass
¼ organic lemon, peeled
2 tsp chopped fresh ginger

In a juicer, process all ingredients.

> *Tip: Add a small slice of lemon to drinks (or squeeze a bit of lemon juice into them) to cut the bitterness of the greens.*

KICK ACID

MAKES 1–2 SERVINGS

This juice is loaded with nutrients and is very alkalinizing. If you're new to juicing greens, go easy on the kale at first and slowly increase the amount over time.

1 head romaine lettuce
4–6 kale leaves
1 whole cucumber
6 celery stalks
½ organic lemon, peeled

In a juicer, process all ingredients and drink immediately.

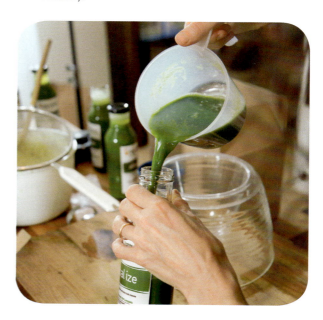

INFLAMMATION BUSTER

MAKES 2 SERVINGS

Sweet, zesty, and juicy, this thirst-quencher will revitalize you when you are tired or stressed. Pineapple contains the enzyme bromelain, known for its anti-inflammatory properties. Commonly used as a digestive aid, bromelain is also believed to benefit the circulatory system. The jalapeño pepper will add an instant morning lift-off!

> *Used as a natural remedy for centuries, ginger is known to combat inflammation and nausea. As children, when we had upset stomachs or colds, we were given home-made ginger tea. To relieve morning sickness during the first trimester of my pregnancy, I often sucked on a piece of peeled ginger.*

½ pineapple, peeled and sliced

2 tsp chopped fresh ginger

1 cup loosely packed cilantro

juice of 1 lime

½-in (1-cm) slice jalapeño pepper, or to taste (optional)

In a juicer, process slices of pineapple, alternating with ginger and cilantro. Add fresh lime juice and jalapeño.

> *Tip: To peel and cut a pineapple, lay it on its side, and begin by cutting off the top and bottom. Stand pineapple upright and, moving from top to bottom, slice off 1-in (2.5-cm) wide sections of peel. Slice into rounds.*

WATERMELON COOLER

MAKES 2 SERVINGS

My favorite summer fruit, watermelons are hydrating, alkaline, and very beneficial to the kidneys. This refreshing drink is bound to cool you off on a hot summer day. I use organic seeded varieties of watermelon and don't bother to remove the seeds. Garnish this drink with a sprig of fresh mint.

▶ *My father was an avid watermelon lover, and we often shared a whole one for dessert! We would play a guessing game of who had the most watermelon seeds hidden on their plate behind the watermelon rinds. Melons are approximately 90 percent liquid and leave the stomach quickly. When eaten with other foods, digestion is delayed and fermentation occurs. That's why we say, "Eat melons alone or leave them alone!"*

▶ **What happened to the seeds?**
Until recently, it was rare to find seedless watermelons. Today, many watermelons grown in North America are seedless—the result of hybridization, which also causes fruit with a higher sugar content. When I was a child, watermelons always had black seeds. We were told that if we swallowed one of these seeds, a watermelon would grow in our stomachs—and spitting them out was part of the fun of eating them! When purchasing watermelons, choose the old-fashioned varieties with seeds, often still sold at farmer's markets.

6 cups (1.5 L) watermelon, peeled, coarsely chopped
¼–½ cup (125 mL) loosely packed fresh mint
juice of ½ lime (approximately 2 tbsp)

In a blender or juicer, blend watermelons until smooth. Add mint and pulse until blended well. Stir in lime juice.

ANTI-ULCER COCKTAIL

MAKES 1–2 SERVINGS

Abundant in vitamin C and sulfur, this juice is very effective in treating ulcers. Add more carrots for a sweeter, more palatable drink.

½ head green cabbage
6 carrots (optional), peeled if not organic

In a juicer, process cabbage and carrots. Drink as fresh as possible.

> *My mother used to suffer from ulcers—most likely caused by all the worrying her rebellious teenagers caused! There were four of us, and we were a wild pack. When her ulcers flared up, my younger brother and I took turns juicing cabbage to help relieve her severe pain. It always worked.*
>
> *Cabbage is rich in S-methylmethionine sulfonium chloride, originally called vitamin U because it inhibits ulceration in the digestive system. In folk medicine, cabbage has been used to treat skin ulcers and ulcers in the digestive tract, and paste made of raw cabbage leaves was also used to reduce acute external inflammation.*

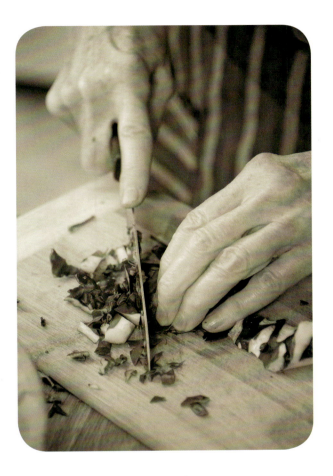

SWEET GREEN MONSTER 🕐

MAKES 1–2 SERVINGS

This is by far the best recipe with which to introduce your family to green smoothies—they won't taste the greens. (If you've never had a green smoothie before, use less romaine and gradually increase the amount as you get used to the taste.)

▶ *Smoothies provide a quick, healthy, and delicious drink that's both nourishing and filling—ideal for rushed mornings. They make great breakfasts or snacks, and are truly the easiest, tastiest way to incorporate more raw fruits and vegetables into your family's diet. Kids love smoothies. Give them a special glass, straw, or spoon to make drinking them more fun!*

2 cups (500 mL) purified water

2 fresh mangos, peeled and chopped

1–2 cups (250–500 mL) roughly chopped romaine lettuce

1 heaping tbsp soaked chia seeds (p. 39)

1 tbsp hemp seeds

In a blender, process all ingredients until smooth.

MY THAI SMOOTHIE 🕐

MAKES 1–2 SERVINGS

Bold, exotic, and flavorful—this drink is a favorite at my SimplyRaw Express restaurant.

2 cups (500 mL) purified water

2 cups (500 mL) peeled and chopped fresh mangos

½ cup (125 mL) loosely packed chopped cilantro

4-in (10-cm) slice cucumber

1 tbsp melted coconut oil

2 tbsp soaked chia seeds (p. 39)

2 tbsp hemp seeds

1 tbsp lime juice

sweetener of choice (optional), to taste

In a blender, process all ingredients until smooth.

STRAWBERRY FIELDS SMOOTHIE

MAKES 1–2 SERVINGS

The ultimate "mylkshake." Over the years, I've fooled many of my son's "fussy eater" friends into believing that this creamy pink shake is made with "normal" ingredients! Be sure to slip in nutritional extras like I do.

2 cups (500 mL) almond (or other non-dairy) mylk

2 cups (500 mL) frozen strawberries

½ banana (fresh or frozen)

2 tbsp hemp seeds

2 tsp melted coconut oil

1 tsp vanilla extract

2–3 pitted soft Medjool dates

In a blender, process all ingredients until smooth.

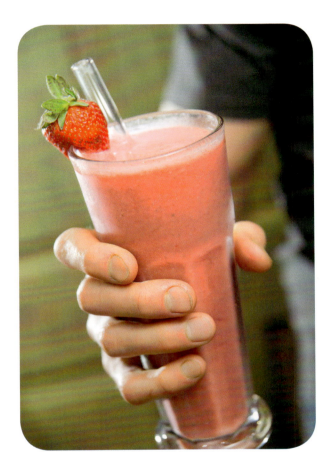

TROPICAL MINT SMOOTHIE

MAKES 1–2 SERVINGS

The combination of pineapple and mint makes this the perfect refreshing drink on a hot summer's day. Pour into a glass and garnish with a few mint leaves.

2 cups (500 mL) purified water

2 cups (500 mL) peeled, chopped pineapple
   (fresh or frozen)

1 frozen banana

6 mint leaves

1 cup (250 mL) packed chopped romaine lettuce

2 tbsp ground dry flax seeds

1 tbsp soaked chia seeds (p. 39)

1 tbsp maple syrup or a few drops stevia (optional)

In a blender, process all ingredients until smooth.

 Adding a frozen banana gives smoothies a creamy texture and natural sweetness.

MANGO LASSI

MAKES 1–2 SERVINGS

This delicious smoothie makes a light, refreshing breakfast, lunch, or dinner. Cardamom is good for the digestion and gives the smoothie a wonderful flavor. Serve this in a tall glass, over ice if you wish.

2 cups (500 mL) nut or seed mylk

2 cups (500 mL) frozen, peeled, and chopped mangos

1 tbsp maple syrup, or to taste

1 whole cardamom pod

1 tsp lemon juice

1 tsp vanilla extract

2 tbsp hemp seeds

1 tbsp soaked chia seeds (p. 39)

In a blender, process all ingredients until smooth.

If you don't have mylk, add 2 tbsp almond butter to recipes that require nut mylk.

SHAMROCK MINT CHIP SHAKE

MAKES 1–2 SERVINGS

Spinach paired with chocolate? Your family will never know that there is a healthy salad hiding in this delicious chocolate shake! Sprinkle a few cacao nibs on top and garnish with a mint sprig before serving.

1½ cups (375 mL) almond mylk

2 large frozen bananas

2 tbsp almond butter

¼ cup (60 mL) packed mint leaves

1 cup (250 mL) packed spinach leaves

1 tsp vanilla extract

2 heaping tbsp raw cacao nibs

In a blender, process all ingredients, except cacao nibs, until smooth. Add nibs, pulsing briefly.

Tip: If you don't have fresh mint leaves, use a drop or two of mint extract.

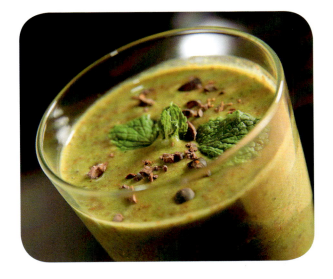

CHOC-O-LOVE SHAKE

MAKES 1–2 SERVINGS

Quite possibly the healthiest, most delicious chocolate shake you will ever drink! Serve it in a tall glass.

1½ cups (375 mL) water

2 large frozen bananas

1 tsp vanilla extract

1–2 cups packed, chopped romaine lettuce

2 tbsp hemp seeds

¼–½ ripe avocado

3 tbsp cacao powder

1–2 tsp maca (optional)

In a blender, process all ingredients until smooth.

▶ *Raw cacao powder is made from unroasted cacao beans and is minimally processed. It's delicious in smoothies, puddings, cakes, frostings, and other chocolate treats. Although cacao is a better choice than traditional chocolate, it does contain caffeine and theobromine. If you can't find raw cacao powder at the natural health food store, use unsweetened cocoa powder.*

▶ *Maca is an ancient Peruvian food that has been used traditionally to enhance fertility and sexual performance in both men and women. It's sold as a powder in most health food stores.*

BASIC NUT OR SEED MYLK

MAKES ABOUT 3 ½ CUPS (830 mL)

Almond or Brazil nut mylk are my personal favorites, since they are amazing sources of antioxidants and protein. To make a great mylk for growing children, use creamy, calcium-rich sesame seeds.

3 cups (750 mL) purified water

1 cup (250 mL) nuts or seeds of choice, soaked and rinsed

In a blender or food processor, process water and nuts or seeds until smooth. Strain mylk through an inside-out (seam-side out) nut mylk bag suspended over a bowl.

▶ *Plain nut and seed mylks keep for 3 days if refrigerated. However, once fruit is added to the mylk, it's best to consume within the day. I usually keep a large sealed Mason jar of plain mylk in the refrigerator.*

SUGAR-KISSED PECAN MYLK

MAKES 4 SERVINGS

Pecan pie in a glass—perfection. This drink is especially good during the fall or winter months, and it can be lightly warmed. Delicious served for dessert or with your favorite healthy cookies.

1 cup (250 mL) pecans, soaked for 8 hours and rinsed

3 cups (750 mL) purified water

3 tbsp maple syrup or a few drops stevia

2 tsp vanilla extract

½ tsp ground cinnamon

⅛ tsp Himalayan salt

1 tbsp coconut oil

In a blender or food processor, process all ingredients until smooth. Strain mixture through a nut mylk bag suspended over a bowl and chill.

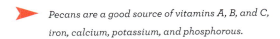 *Pecans are a good source of vitamins A, B, and C, iron, calcium, potassium, and phosphorous.*

ONE-MINUTE MIRACLE MYLK

MAKES 1 SERVING

Nothing beats fresh almond mylk! If you don't have almonds in the house, get out that jar of almond butter (or other nut/seed butter of choice) and start blending. What could be easier?

1–2 heaping tbsp raw almond butter

1 cup (250 mL) purified water

1 tsp maple syrup (optional)

½ tsp vanilla extract or ground cinnamon (optional)

In a blender process all ingredients until creamy.

▶ *Almonds are a rich source of manganese, magnesium, and vitamin E, which can help reduce the risk of heart disease. They are high in monounsaturated fats, which play a role in lowering LDL-cholesterol. Studies have also shown that, when eaten with a meal, almonds can lower its glycemic index, providing extra protection against diabetes.*

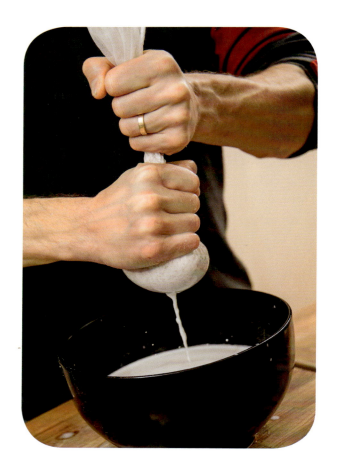

VANILLA ALMOND MYLK

MAKES 1 QT (1 L)

A creamy, slightly sweet mylk to drink alone, in smoothies, or over cereal—without clogging up your precious
arteries. You will never go back to dairy again! Adjust
the sweetness to taste, and if you prefer a lower fat,
"skim" mylk, simply use more water. A pinch of salt
brings out the flavor but is entirely optional.

1 cup (250 mL) almonds, soaked overnight and rinsed
3 cups (750 mL) purified water
3–4 dates or 3 tbsp (60 mL) maple syrup or a few
    drops stevia (optional)
1 tbsp vanilla extract or ½ tsp ground vanilla bean
⅛ tsp Himalayan salt (optional)

In a blender or food processor, process all ingredients
on high until creamy. Strain through a nut mylk bag
suspended over a bowl. (You can skip this step if you
want the fiber, but I strongly suggest straining, especially if you're making this for children.)

Vanilla extract is a delicious, aromatic flavoring that brings a whole new level of taste to desserts and smoothies. I prefer the alcohol-free kind, but if you can't find it, use vanilla beans or vanilla bean powder. You can make alcohol-free vanilla extract by blending three chopped vanilla beans with 1 cup (250 mL) purified water. It will keep, if refrigerated, for about 1 month.

Variations:

Chocolate Mylk: Use the recipe for Vanilla Almond Mylk, and add 2–4 tbsp raw cacao nibs or unsweetened raw cacao powder.

Cinnamon Mylk: Use the recipe for Vanilla Almond Mylk, and add 1 tsp ground cinnamon and ⅛ tsp ground nutmeg.

Chai Mylk: Use the recipe for Vanilla Almond Milk, and add 1 tsp ground cinnamon, ½ tsp ground ginger, ½ teaspoon garam masala, and ¼ tsp ground nutmeg.

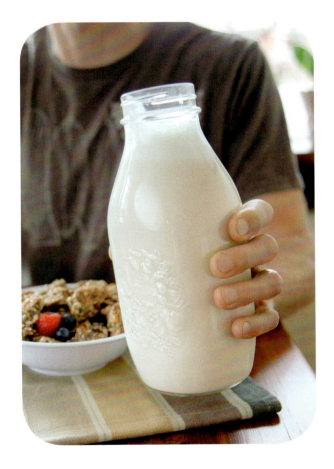

INSTANT HEMP MYLK

MAKES 2 SERVINGS

Unlike most other seeds and nuts, hemp seeds don't need to be soaked or strained, so they're perfect for rushed mornings!

½ cup (125 mL) hemp seeds
2 cups (500 mL) purified water
2 tsp maple syrup
dash Himalayan salt
½ tsp vanilla extract

In a blender or food processor, process all ingredients until smooth. Either chill before serving or use cold water or an ice cube or piece of frozen fruit.

> *Also called hemp hearts, hemp seeds are an extraordinary source of omega-3 fatty acids as well as a complete protein. Hemp seeds can be added to smoothies, soups, and salads for an extra boost of nutrition.*

DO-IT-YOURSELF COCONUT MYLK

MAKES ABOUT 3½ CUPS (830 mL)

A delicious beverage that doesn't require a can opener or machete! It makes a great base in smoothies, soups, and sauces.

2 cups (500 mL) organic dried and unsweetened
    coconut flakes
3 cups (750 mL) very warm water
⅛ tsp Himalayan salt (optional)
1 tsp vanilla extract (optional)

In a large bowl, soak coconut flakes in water for 20–30 minutes. (You can skip this step if you're in a rush.) Transfer mixture to blender. In blender, add salt and vanilla and blend until creamy (approximately 2–3 minutes). Strain through a nut mylk bag suspended over a bowl. Save pulp for dehydrating or baking. Store mylk in a glass container in refrigerator for up to 3 days. Give it a good shake if separation occurs.

> *Canned foods often contain added sodium and preservatives. Cans themselves may also leach Bisphenol-A (BPA) into the food.*

About Thai Coconuts

The Thai coconut in its natural state is young and green, but when sold at Asian markets, it often appears white with a conical top. Inside is the soft coconut "meat" and coconut water.

The first time I tasted a young coconut was in 1986 when I lived on a coconut plantation in Thailand. It was fresh off the tree, and I fell in love! I drank coconut water each and every day thereafter, climbing up trees to fetch my own—to the amusement of my Thai friends. When I returned to Canada, my love affair continued. I would balance cases of Thai coconuts on my bicycle as I brought them home from Chinatown. I was also the talk of the apartment building as I husked young coconuts on my balcony with my shiny long machete.

Since learning that Thai coconuts are treated with chemicals to sanitize them before exporting, I now use them less frequently—unless they're organic. I've also discovered a simple way to prepare my own coconut mylk using shredded coconut flakes and water (see p. 64). Although nowhere near as tasty or nutritious as the real thing, homemade coconut mylk adds flavor to smoothies, raw desserts, soups, and sauces.

Coconut water is a clear, hydrating liquid that comes from the inside of the young coconut. Particularly rich in the potassium, coconut water has recently been recognized as "nature's sport drink," as it contains a variety of trace elements, vitamins, minerals, and amino acids, and is very alkaline. I have done many fasts during which I drank only coconut water and wheatgrass juice.

Coconut water has traditionally been used to treat digestive disturbances, bladder infections, diarrhea, kidney stones, circulatory problems, and high blood pressure.

VANILLA BEAN BUBBLE MYLK

MAKES 4 SERVINGS

A bubble tea that is rich in nutrients without processed sugars or food colorings. Make it in the evening to allow time for the chia to expand overnight.
This is truly delicious!

3 cups (750 mL) almond mylk

⅛ tsp Himalayan salt (optional)

1 tsp vanilla powder or 1 tbsp vanilla extract

3 tbsp maple syrup

2 tbsp melted coconut oil

3 tbsp soaked chia seeds (p. 39)

In a blender, process all ingredients except chia seeds
until smooth. Transfer to a mason jar and add chia,
stirring thoroughly to prevent clumping. Seal jar and
refrigerate for 30 minutes. Shake periodically.

➤ *An ancient food, chia is a nutritional powerhouse*
loaded with vitamins, minerals, protein, and
antioxidants. Chia seeds are a rich source
of omega-3 fatty acids and are excellent in
smoothies, puddings, soups, crackers, and
desserts. Always soak chia before eating for
optimal bio-availability. Aztec legend says
that their warriors and runners could sustain
themselves for an entire day on just one
tablespoon of chia seeds.

Variation: Use Brazil nut mylk for a selenium-rich drink.

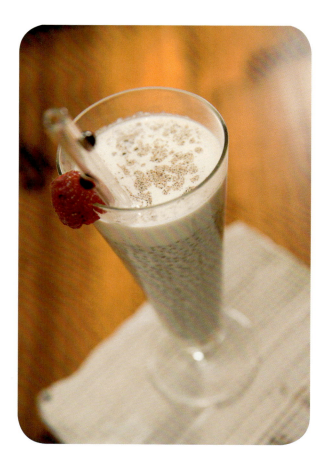

YOGI TEA

MAKES 1.5 G (6 L)

I lived through many Canadian winters without consuming anything heated. Since turning fifty, I find that my body feels better when some warming foods are included in my diet. I was first introduced to Yogi Tea in 1995 by Siri Bandhu, my prenatal yoga teacher and proprietor of Vegy B&B in Ottawa (vegybnb. com). Her house always smelled deliciously of this divine tea. I find this drink warming and invigorating. It can be made in advance and stored in the refrigerator for several days. **Tip:** Spices can be reused once.

1.5 g (6 L) purified water
1 tbsp whole cloves
32 whole cardamom pods
1 tbsp black peppercorns
8 6-in (15-cm) sticks of cinnamon
8-in (20-cm) slice thick fresh ginger
2 jasmine (or green) tea bags

In a large stainless steel pot on high, bring all ingredients to a boil. Reduce heat to medium and simmer for 5 minutes. Reduce heat to low, cover pot, and simmer for 40 minutes, until aromatic. Remove from heat. Strain as soon as tea has cooled enough to handle. Sweeten to taste and/or add almond mylk for a warming winter treat. Store in refrigerator.

Variation: Add 1 tbsp or more fennel seeds to make tea somewhat diuretic and give it a sweeter flavor.

Yogi tea was popularized by Yogi Bhajan, an Indian spiritual teacher who also introduced Kundalini yoga to the US in 1969. After each yoga class, his special spice tea was served to his students, which they affectionately named Yogi Tea. An Ayurvedic blend of five traditional spices, it is a tonic drink that is said to stimulate the immune system, aid digestion, and increase vitality.

Yogi Bhajan described the ingredients: "Cloves take away pain, cardamom aids digestion, cinnamon is good for the bones, black pepper stimulates the digestive process, and ginger is an Ayurvedic panacea, giving strength and energy. And the synergistic effect of all the herbs is more than the sum of its parts."

SUN TEA

MAKES 6 SERVINGS

Made by infusing loose tea leaves or other herbs in water for several hours under the natural heat of the sun, this tea makes a refreshing beverage. Although the process is simple, it does require patience—especially if you're living in a Northern climate!

¼–⅓ cup (60–80 mL) dried herbs (or ½–1 cup [125–250 mL] fresh)

2 qt (2 L) purified water

In a large Mason jar, combine herbs and water. Place in a sunny location, in- or outdoors. After about 4 hours, strain tea. Chill if desired. The longer the tea sits in the sun, the more flavorful it will be.

 Try combining two or more different types of herbs to create a blend. Add orange or lemon zest.

HOLIDAY NUT NOG

MAKES 3 SERVINGS

A luxurious, velvety drink to share with loved ones at Christmas and throughout the year. You will never miss dairy or soy nog again!

4 cups (1 L) almond mylk

2 heaping tbsp chia seeds, soaked for 4–6 hours

1 tbsp melted coconut oil

1 tsp ground nutmeg

1 tsp ground cinnamon

1 tbsp vanilla extract or ¼ tsp vanilla powder

⅛ tsp Himalayan salt

⅛ tsp turmeric (optional, for color)

2 frozen bananas

½ tsp grated nutmeg, for garnish

In blender, process all ingredients, except bananas and nutmeg, until creamy. Refrigerate until serving. Just before serving, add bananas and blend until smooth. Serve chilled.

 *Vanilla powder is derived from the orchid plant **V. planifolia**. It tends to be quite pricey, but brings a depth of flavor to drinks and desserts. If you don't have powder, use alcohol-free vanilla extract or a piece of vanilla bean. Some recipes call for scraping the vanilla seeds from the inside of the bean and then discarding the rest. This is a waste—the entire vanilla bean is filled with flavor!*

WARMED WHITE CHOCOLATE

MAKES 2 SERVINGS

Sometimes, a rich cup of creamy white cocoa is all you need!

1½ cups (375 mL) warm water

1 cup (250 mL) cashews, soaked in 2 cups (500 mL) water for 30 minutes or more

¼ cup (60 mL) grated raw cacao butter

1 tsp vanilla extract

3 tbsp maple syrup

dash Himalayan salt

1 tbsp melted coconut oil

½ tsp cacao powder, for garnish

In a blender, process all ingredients until smooth. Pour into 2 mugs and sprinkle with cacao powder.

▶ *High in fat, cacao butter makes amazing chocolate when mixed with cacao. It is sold in solid form. To melt, grate into a bowl. Cover and place in a bowl of hot water or on top of running dehydrator.*

▶ *Raw cashews are naturally sweet and lend a smooth, creamy quality to mylks, cheezes, and dressings. Soak cashews (for 30 minutes to 2 hours) before using in most recipes. Because cashews are soft, there's no need to strain them through a nut mylk bag.*

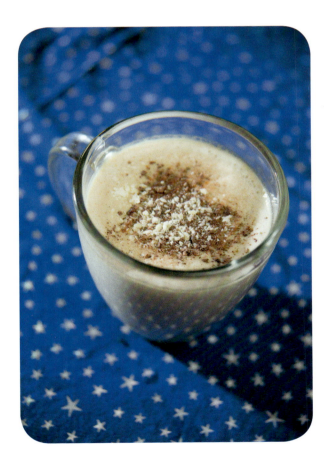

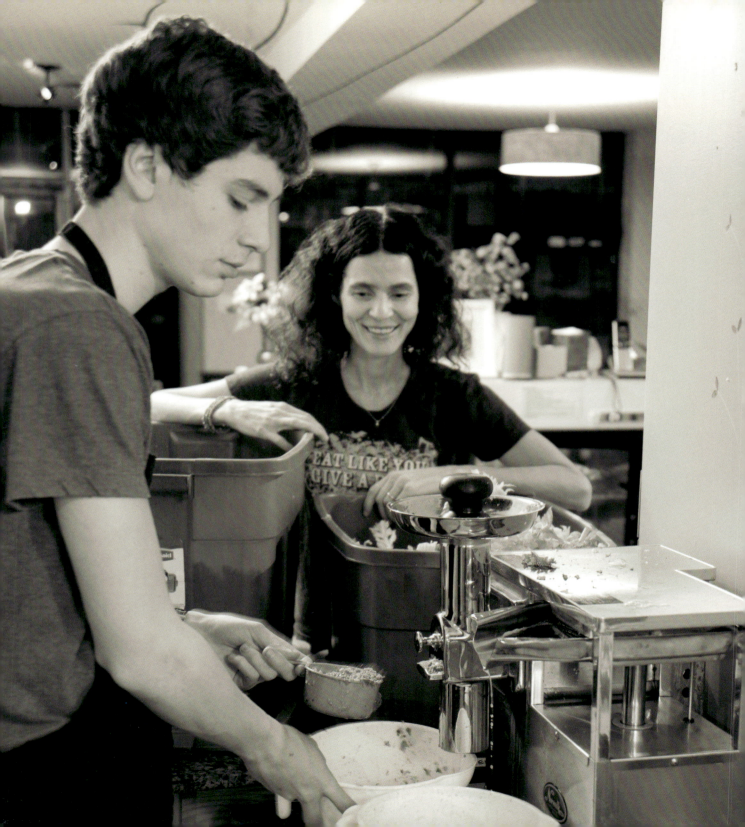

BREAKFASTS

Spiced Chia Tapioca 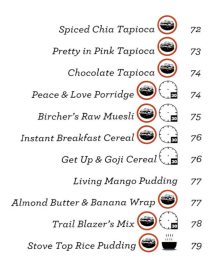 72

Pretty in Pink Tapioca 73

Chocolate Tapioca 74

Peace & Love Porridge 74

Bircher's Raw Muesli 75

Instant Breakfast Cereal 76

Get Up & Goji Cereal 76

Living Mango Pudding 77

Almond Butter & Banana Wrap 77

Trail Blazer's Mix 78

Stove Top Rice Pudding 79

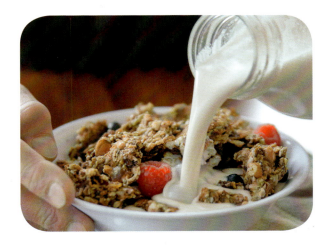

One of the easiest ways to include fresh fruits and vegetables in your diet is to start the day with a nutrient-packed breakfast. A healthy meal in the morning sets the tone for the rest for the day, and a breakfast of fresh plant foods will result in higher energy levels and greater clarity.

Like many raw foodists, I prefer to "break my fast" with something juicy and easy on the digestion. I greet my mornings with plenty of water, an ounce or two of wheatgrass, and a tall glass of green juice or a smoothie. For me, this approach works best.

In the winter season, however, many of us desire a heartier and more substantial breakfast; greens are often followed with a raw cereal to provide our bodies with long-lasting energy.

The following breakfast options are simple, satisfying, and nourishing, prepared with fruit, nuts, seeds, and whole, gluten-free grains—healthy alternatives to the standard boxed cereals that offer little nutritional value. They can be enjoyed with nut mylk in the morning, at lunch, as a snack, or any time throughout the day.

SPICED CHIA TAPIOCA

MAKES 4 SERVINGS

Packed with nutrition, chia seeds should be included in our daily diets. Make this pudding the night before so that a deeply nourishing breakfast awaits you in the morning. Serve drizzled with maple syrup or topped diced apples and dusted with cinnamon. (To make a nut-free version, use sesame or coconut mylk.)

2 cups (500 mL) almond mylk (or mylk of choice)
2 tbsp hemp seeds
1½ tsp ground cinnamon
¼ tsp ground nutmeg
½ tsp ground ginger
3–4 tbsp maple syrup
¼ cup (60 mL) unsoaked chia seeds

In a blender on low, process all ingredients except chia seeds. Pour into a Mason jar and add chia. Stir with a whisk or fork to remove clumps. Seal jar. Shake several times over the next 20 minutes. Refrigerate and allow to thicken for at least 2 hours, preferably overnight. Tapioca will keep for about 5–7 days if refrigerated.

PRETTY IN PINK TAPIOCA

MAKES 4 SERVINGS

This chia pudding, reminiscent of tapioca, is the best I've ever tasted; it makes a great introduction to chia seeds for children.

1 cup (250 mL) almond mylk (or milk of choice)
1 cup (250 mL) raspberries, fresh or frozen and
    thawed
2 tbsp hemp seeds
1 tbsp melted coconut oil
1 tsp vanilla extract
3–4 tbsp maple syrup
¼ cup (60 mL) unsoaked chia seeds

In a blender on low speed, combine all ingredients except chia. Pour into Mason jar and add chia seeds. Stir with a whisk or fork to remove clumps. Seal jar. Shake several times over next 20 minutes. Refrigerate and allow to thicken for at least 2 hours, preferably overnight. Tapioca will keep for approximately 5–7 days refrigerated.

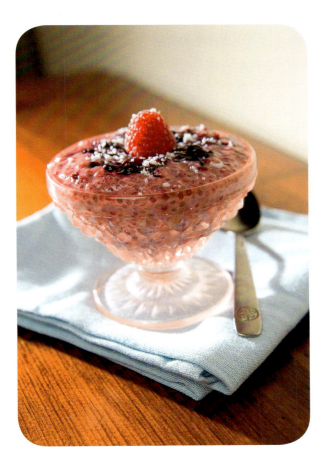

CHOCOLATE TAPIOCA

MAKES 4–6 SERVINGS

It's hard to believe that something so rich and tasty can be good for you—especially for breakfast! Using carob powder instead of cacao makes it even healthier!

2 cups (500 mL) Brazil nut mylk

2 tbsp cacao or carob powder

1 tsp vanilla extract

¼ tsp ground cinnamon

¼ cup (60 mL) maple syrup

2 tbsp hemp seeds

1 tsp melted coconut oil

¼ cup (60 mL) unsoaked chia seeds

In a Mason jar, combine all ingredients. Stir to remove clumps. Seal jar. Shake several times over the next 20 minutes. Refrigerate. Allow to thicken for at least 2 hours, preferably overnight.

➤ *Carob comes from the carob bean. It has a naturally sweet taste but, unlike chocolate, it doesn't contain caffeine, theobromine, or oxalic acid; it's also lower in fat. Substitute carob for chocolate (or use half and half) in smoothies, shakes, and desserts.*

PEACE & LOVE PORRIDGE

MAKES 2 SERVINGS

A popular Russian staple made from cooked buckwheat, this hearty raw porridge will rock the kasha! Top with berries and additional cinnamon or shredded coconut, nuts, and seeds.

2 cups (500 mL) soaked buckwheat groats (see p. 39)

¼ cup (60 mL) hemp seeds

2 fresh bananas

1 cup (250 mL) almond mylk (or mylk of choice)

2 tsp vanilla extract

1 tbsp melted coconut oil

1–2 tbsp maple syrup or a few drops vanilla stevia (optional)

1 tsp ground cinnamon (optional)

⅛ tsp ground nutmeg

½ cup (125 mL) Thompson raisins

In a blender or food processor, blend all ingredients except raisins until slightly smooth. Add raisins and pulse briefly.

➤ *Buckwheat is not related to wheat, nor is it a grain, but a fruit seed botanically related to rhubarb. It is highly nutritious, rich in B vitamins, iron, and selenium. Buckwheat is gluten-free and makes a nutritious substitute for wheat or grains. Kasha is porridge made from buckwheat groats.*

BIRCHER'S RAW MUESLI

MAKES 2 SERVINGS

My Austrian mother often fed us muesli before we ran off to school. This is a delicious, mainly raw version (the rolled oats are heated). Use gluten-free certified oats if you have sensitivities.

 As legend goes, muesli was invented around 1900 by physician Maximilian Bircher-Benner as a nutritious breakfast for patients in his Swiss hospital. Dr Bircher-Benner encouraged his patients to eat less bread and meat and more nuts, vegetables, and fruit. He promoted physical exercise and fresh air, and his patients spent time gardening every day. Their regimen was modeled on Bircher-Benner's conception of the daily lives of Swiss shepherds.

1 cup (250 mL) rolled oats

¼ cup (60 mL) coarsely chopped dry raw almonds

1 apple, grated

¼ cup (60 mL) goji berries

¼ cup (60 mL) raisins

2 tbsp soaked chia seeds (p. 39)

1½ cups (375 mL) almond or mylk of choice

dash salt (optional)

about ½ cup (125 mL) fresh blueberries (optional, but delicious)

1–2 tsp maple syrup (optional)

In a large bowl, place all ingredients except blueberries and maple syrup and soak overnight. Top with blueberries and a dash of maple syrup before serving.

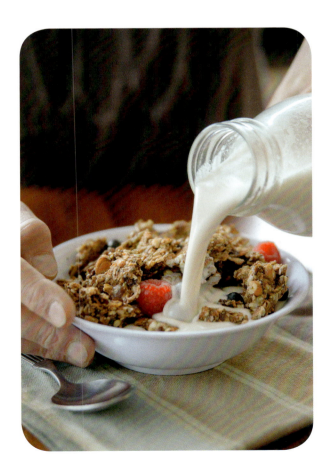

INSTANT BREAKFAST CEREAL

MAKES 1 SERVING

A healthy quick breakfast, ideal for winter mornings. Drizzle with a touch of maple syrup or a few drops of stevia, if desired, and top with your favorite mylk.

1 apple, chopped

2 tbsp Thompson raisins

2 tbsp hemp seeds

¼ cup (60 mL) almonds, soaked overnight

2 tbsp sunflower seed, soaked overnight

2 tbsp soaked and sprouted buckwheat groats

½ tsp ground cinnamon

Rinse and drain nuts and seeds. In a serving bowl, combine all ingredients, mixing thoroughly.

GET UP & GOJI CEREAL

MAKES 2 SERVINGS

A nutrient-dense, nut-free cereal that will keep you energized all morning long. Goji berries are an excellent source of antioxidants and vitamin C; hemp is rich in healthy omegas and protein; and pumpkin seeds are high in zinc, magnesium, and iron. Top with your favorite mylk and a handful of fresh blueberries or some banana slices, and sweeten to taste.

➤ *If you have a dehydrator, you can soak and dehydrate batches of nuts and seeds in advance—these are great to have ready on hand for quick(er) breakfasts.*

1 apple, cored and chopped

¼ cup (60 mL) pumpkin seeds, soaked overnight

¼ cup (60 mL) sunflower seeds, soaked overnight

2 tbsp hemp seeds

¼ cup (60 mL) coconut flakes

¼ cup (60 mL) goji berries

¼ cup (60 mL) Thompson raisins

¼ tsp ground cinnamon

dash Himalayan salt

Rinse and drain soaked pumpkin and sunflower seeds. In a food processor, blend seeds with remainder of ingredients and pulse briefly to mix.

LIVING MANGO PUDDING

MAKES 2 SERVINGS

There is nothing better than a simple, nutritious breakfast. This is one of them.

2 mangos, peeled and chopped
1 fresh ripe banana
2 tbsp hemp seeds
about ½ cup (125 mL) sunflower sprouts

In a blender, process all ingredients until smooth. Pour into a bowl and enjoy.

ALMOND BUTTER & BANANA WRAP

MAKES 1 SERVING

I love this version of fast food. Grab a leaf, peel a banana, spread some almond butter, and wrap it up for breakfast on the go!

1 tbsp almond butter
1 banana
1 large kale or collard leaf
sweetener of choice (optional)

Spread almond butter into crease of kale leaf and drizzle with a touch of sweetener if desired. Place whole, peeled banana in center of leaf and wrap.

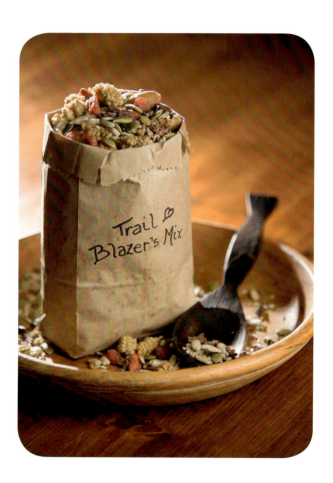

> Hailed as the latest superfood, goji berries are high in antioxidants and packed with vitamin C and beta carotene.

TRAIL BLAZER'S MIX

MAKES 4–6 SERVINGS

Just a few handfuls of this super-nutritious trail mix will provide your body with enough energy to keep you going for hours. Keep a container of it handy in your purse, knapsack, lunch box, or glove compartment. You can add your own favorite ingredients to it— almost anything goes!

½ cup (125 mL) goji berries

½ cup (125 mL) cacao nibs

½ cup (125 mL) sunflower seeds, soaked and dehydrated

½ cup (125 mL) pumpkin seeds, soaked and dehydrated

½ cup (125 mL) Brazil nuts, soaked and dehydrated

¼ cup (60 mL) hemp seeds

½ cup (125 mL) mulberries

In a large bowl, combine all ingredients.

> Mulberries are a chewy dried fruit that makes a tasty nutritious snack. They are an excellent source of vitamin C, calcium, fiber, protein, and iron. Mulberries also contain the polyphenol resveratrol, a powerful antioxidant that can help lower cholesterol.

STOVETOP RICE PUDDING

MAKES 2–3 SERVINGS

Sweet and creamy, rice pudding served hot or cold is a comforting treat for young and old. Eat it plain, with a dusting of cinnamon, or garnished with fresh berries.

3 cups (750 mL) purified water

½ cup (125 mL) short-grain brown rice

⅛ tsp Himalayan salt

2 cups (500 mL) almond mylk

1 tsp ground cardamom seeds

⅛ tsp ground cloves

⅛ tsp ground cinnamon

1 tsp grated fresh ginger or ¼ tsp ground ginger

¼ cup (60 mL) maple syrup

⅛ tsp ground nutmeg

1 tbsp grated orange rind

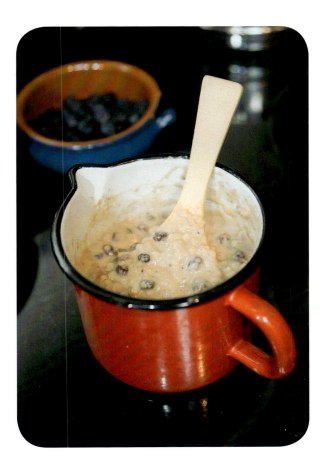

In a medium saucepan on high, bring water with rice and salt to a boil. Reduce heat to medium, cover saucepan, and stir occasionally for 50 minutes, until water is almost absorbed. Gradually add almond mylk, stirring constantly as the pudding becomes sticky and creamy. Cook for 20 minutes; add remainder of ingredients in last 5 minutes. Remove saucepan from heat, cover, and let sit for another 20 minutes. Stir before serving.

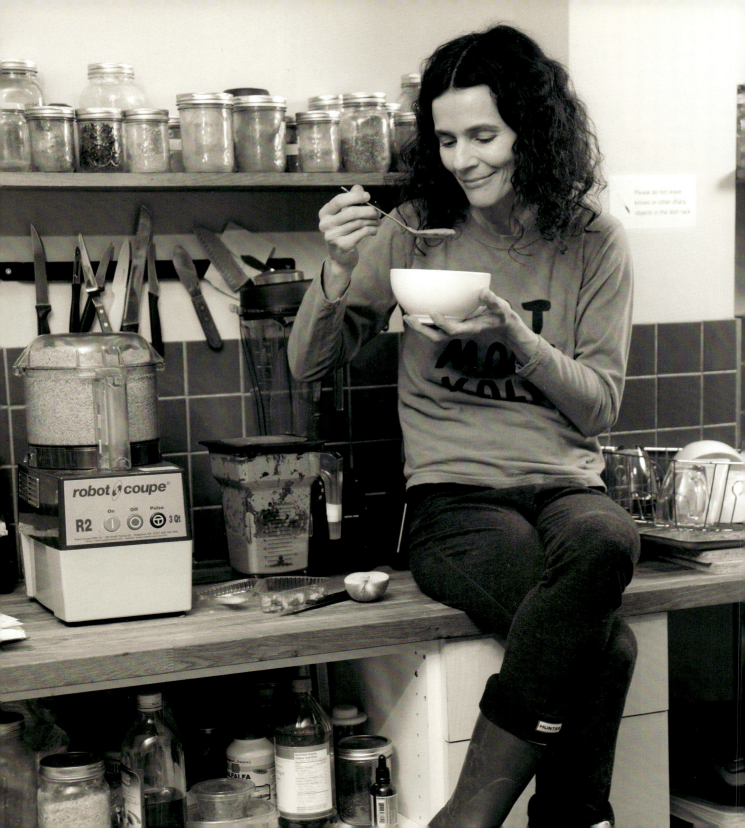

SOUPS

Light Garden Blend	83
Thom Kha Soup	84
Popeye Soup	85
Real Tomato Soup	86
Sweet Corn Chowder	88
Green Curry Soup	90
Spicy Mexican Lime Soup	91
Creamy Zucchini Bisque	92
Alkaline Mineral Broth	93
Soup Stock	94
Wild Garlic (or Leek) Soup	95
About Garlic	96
Tomato-Millet Soup	97
Babuschka's Borscht	98
Cauliflower Chowder	100
Lentil Soup with Kale	101
About Miso	102
Miso Soup with Shiitake Mushrooms	103

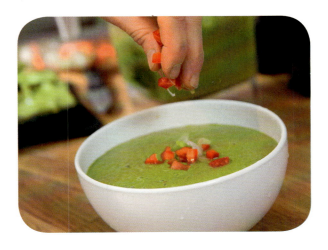

No food says "comfort" more than soup. As ancient as cooking itself, and once considered humble peasant food, an appetizing bowl of soup is a welcome addition to any table. A great soup is satisfying, pleasing to the palate, and has the power to lift our spirits and nourish our souls. Raw or cooked, hot or cold, spicy or mild, there's a revitalizing bowl for every need.

Soups made a regular appearance at meal times when I was growing up; my mother would make use of whatever vegetables were in season. She could make any soup taste amazing simply by adding a pinch of this or a touch of that. Potatoes, squash, carrots, onions, and tomatoes with herbs were added to a pot of water or stock on the stove to create a gratifying, hearty, and nutritious lunch, perfectly paired with a slice of dark rye bread. Soup was not just the first course—it was the meal. It always brings me back to my childhood—sitting in front of a warm oven enjoying a hot bowl on a cold winter day.

As a raw foodist, I now prepare my own entirely satisfying, soul-warming, but uncooked soups that are versatile and nutritious. Since most raw soups are made using a blender, they are convenient, easy to put together, and—an added bonus!—require little cleanup. Raw soups are just as satisfying as their cooked counterparts. You can make some real magic happen in a blender with just the right balance of flavors and by using fresh organic produce of the highest quality.

No matter what the season, I enjoy having soup almost every day, especially as part of my evening meal when I need something more soothing than salad. In colder weather or climates, you may want to warm raw soups lightly on the stove or in the dehydrator, or use hot water instead of cold.

Soups are a quick and convenient way to provide your body with plenty of easily digestible fiber, protein, vitamins, and minerals. Because raw soups are blended, it is easier to extract the nutrients from the vegetables with very little time or digestive effort. They are also low in fat and sodium. Serve soups with dehydrated crackers, a slice of gluten-free bread, or—my favorite—crispy, easy-to-digest romaine hearts to dip into them.

The secret to making a good raw soup is to blend a mix of vegetables with water or another liquid, a fat for creaminess, something salty, herbs for seasoning (fresh if possible), and a bit of acidity, to balance all the flavors. Because I love spicy foods, cayenne or some other pepper is also a common ingredient in my soups. Occasionally, I'll add a small piece of fruit (apple, orange, mango) to give the soup a natural sweetness. I prefer to keep soup as simple as possible, but feel free to adjust flavorings to your tastes in the recipes that follow.

I encourage you to use organic ingredients. Experiment with different vegetables and herbs; taste as you go, and be adventurous—you'll be surprised how delicious and easy raw soups can be.

> *My mother insists that soup—whether raw or cooked—is not complete without a green garnish (parsley, dill, cilantro, basil).*

LIGHT GARDEN BLEND

MAKES 2–4 SERVINGS

A delicate, light soup with the refreshing flavor of dill.

¼ medium red onion, roughly chopped

4 cups (1 L) roughly chopped celery

2 cups (500 mL) peeled and roughly chopped zucchini

2 cups (500 mL) chopped romaine lettuce

2 tbsp lemon juice

1 tsp salt

1 tsp onion powder

1 tbsp gluten-free tamari

⅛ tsp cayenne pepper

½ avocado, chopped

¼ cup (60 mL) chopped fresh dill

In a blender, process 2 cups (500 mL) purified water with all ingredients, except avocado and dill, until smooth. Add avocado and blend again. Garnish with chopped dill.

Variation: Replace dill with your favorite herb or omit altogether.

You may substitute dried herbs for fresh, but because dried herbs are more concentrated, you can use less. A general rule is to substitute 1 tsp dried for every 1 tbsp fresh herbs. Always taste as you go along, and remember that it is easier to add than to subtract seasonings.

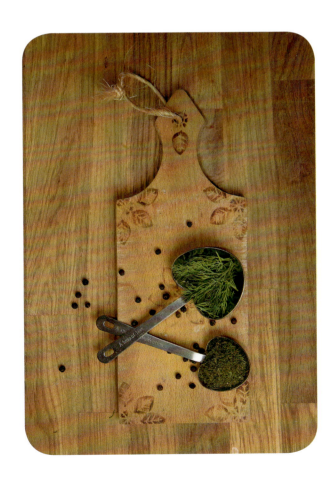

THOM KHA SOUP

MAKES 4 SERVINGS

When I returned to Canada after living in Thailand for a year and began to eat raw, I created this version of my old tropical favorite. If you have access to fresh organic coconuts, blend 2 coconuts with 2 cups coconut water for your soup base. The lemongrass, ginger, and kaffir lime leaves lend this soup a fragrant, Thai-inspired flavor. *Aroy dee!*

4 cups (1 L) shredded organic coconut

2 tbsp lime juice

½ cup (125 mL) chopped lemongrass

2 tbsp maple syrup

½ Thai chili or ½ tsp red pepper flakes

1 tsp Himalayan salt

1 tsp gluten-free tamari

2 tsp chopped fresh ginger

4 kaffir lime leaves

¼ cup (60 mL) finely chopped bok choy or spinach, for garnish

¼ cup (60 mL) diced tomatoes, for garnish

2 tbsp sliced green onions, for garnish

2 tbsp chopped fresh cilantro, for garnish

In a blender, process coconut, 4 cups (1 L) purified hot water, lime juice, lemongrass, maple syrup, chili, salt, tamari, ginger, and kaffir lime leaves until smooth. Strain through a nut mylk bag. *Be careful not to burn your fingers—the liquid will be hot!*

Pour into 4 serving bowls and garnish with bok choy, tomatoes, green onions, and cilantro.

➤ *Kaffir lime leaves can be found in the produce section of most Chinese or Indian grocery stores. The leaves have a strong flavor, so use them sparingly.*

POPEYE SOUP

MAKES 2–4 SERVINGS

My ever-faithful, go-to soup—rich in color and phyto-nutrients. Popeye never had it so healthy!

½ organic apple, cored, unpeeled

1 bunch spinach, about 4 packed cups (1 L)

2 celery stalks

½ red bell pepper, seeded

1 green onion

1 garlic clove (optional)

2 tbsp lemon juice

1 tbsp light miso

1 tbsp raw tahini

1 tbsp gluten-free tamari

dash cayenne pepper, to taste

½ cup (125 mL) fresh cilantro

1 avocado, chopped

2 tbsp sliced green onions, for garnish (optional)

2 tbsp diced red bell pepper, for garnish (optional)

2 tsp hemp seeds, for garnish (optional)

In a blender, process 2 cups (500 mL) purified water, apple, spinach, celery, bell peppers, green onion, garlic, lemon juice, miso, tahini, tamari, cayenne pepper, and cilantro until smooth. Add avocado and blend again. Season to taste. Top with garnishes and serve.

Spinach is a good source of vitamins A B, C, and E, calcium and iron, and several vital antioxidants. However, spinach is one of the "dirty dozen" (produce with heavy pesticide residues) listed by the Environmental Working Group (see p. 27), so buy it organically grown!

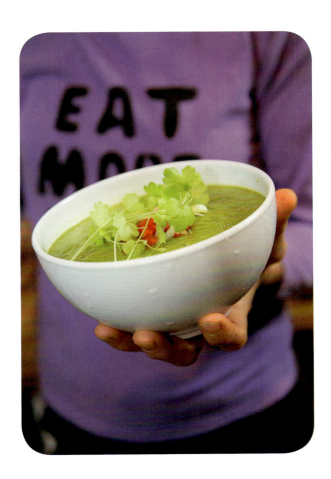

REAL TOMATO SOUP

Delicious, satisfying, and nostalgic. After making this, you will never buy tomato soup in a can again!

MAKES 2–4 SERVINGS

4 large tomatoes, chopped

2 red bell peppers, chopped

½ cup (125 mL) hemp seeds

2 tbsp lime juice

1 tbsp light miso

2 tbsp gluten-free tamari

½ avocado, chopped

1 tbsp maple syrup or a few drops stevia (optional)

dash Himalayan salt, to taste

dash freshly ground black pepper, to taste

2 tbsp chopped chives, for garnish (optional)

In a blender, process tomatoes, bell peppers, hemp seeds, lime juice, miso, tamari, avocado, and maple syrup until smooth. Season to taste and garnish with chives.

▶ **Note**: *Tamari is a "cooked" food. A naturally fermented soy sauce that contains no preservatives or sugar, it adds a rich and salty flavor to dishes (you may choose to use a reduced-sodium variety). Most tamari contains wheat, so look for gluten-free.*

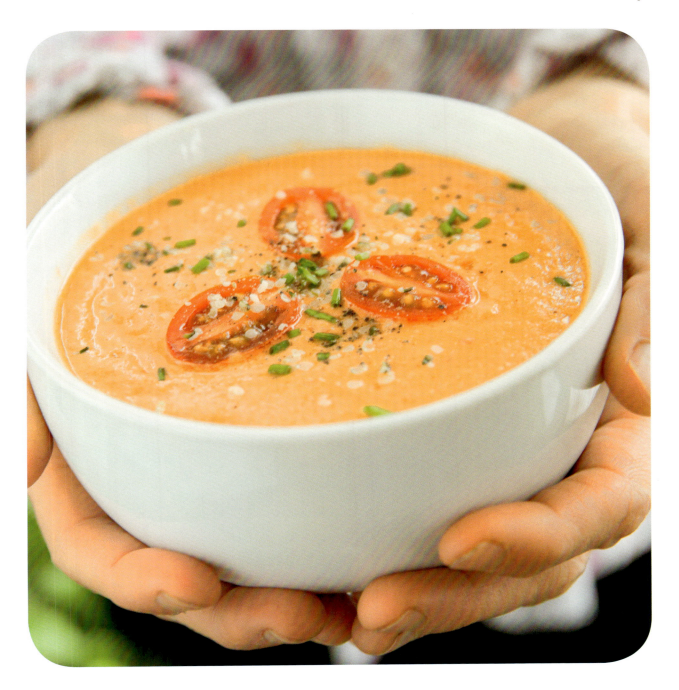

SWEET CORN CHOWDER

Rich and creamy, a bowl of this classic soup brings instant comfort to your table. Serve with dehydrated crackers, guacamole, or Soft Taco Verde (p. 162). For a nut-free, lighter version, replace walnuts with half an avocado.

MAKES 3–4 SERVINGS

½ cup (125 mL) walnuts, soaked for 8 hours

3 cups (750 mL) corn, fresh or frozen

1 cup (250 mL) diced orange bell peppers

1 tsp Himalayan salt, or to taste

2 tbsp gluten-free tamari

3 tbsp fresh lime juice

½ small jalapeño pepper, seeded and deveined (optional)

⅛ tsp freshly ground black pepper

1 tbsp extra virgin olive oil

½ cup (125 mL) lightly packed chopped fresh cilantro

1 cup (125 mL) corn kernels, for garnish

½ avocado, diced, for garnish

¼ cup (60 mL) fresh cilantro leaves, chopped finely, for garnish

In a blender, process 1½ cups (375 mL) purified water (warm, if you prefer) with walnuts until creamy. Add remainder of ingredients except garnishes in order, blending until smooth. Season to taste and top with garnishes.

➤ *Conventionally grown corn may have been genetically modified. There's no requirement to label GM foods in North America, but you can avoid them by purchasing organically grown foods*

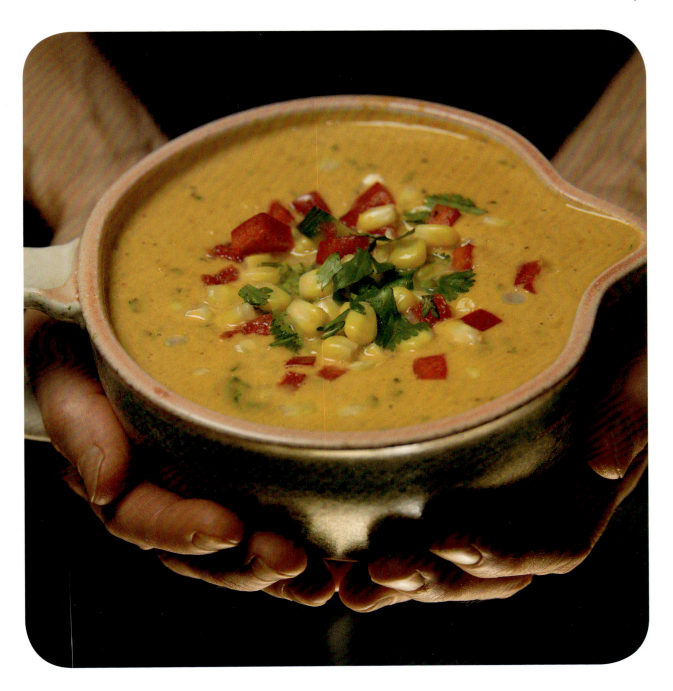

GREEN CURRY SOUP

MAKES 2–4 SERVINGS

This aromatic soup is chock-full of warming spices—making it ideal to serve when the weather's cold. Of course, it's also delicious during the summer, served chilled.

1 garlic clove

¼ cup (60 mL) roughly chopped red onions

2 tsp grated ginger

3 cups (750 mL) chopped, peeled zucchini (approximately 2 large zucchinis)

1 cup (250 mL) chopped, packed spinach

2 tsp lime juice

1 tsp Himalayan salt

1 tbsp gluten-free tamari

1½ tsp ground curry

⅛ tsp ground turmeric

cayenne pepper, to taste

1 avocado, chopped

1 tbsp melted coconut oil

¼ cup (60 mL) chopped cilantro, for garnish

In a blender, blend 2 cups (500 mL) purified water with garlic, onions, and ginger. Add zucchini, spinach, lime juice, salt, tamari, and spices and blend until smooth. Add avocado and coconut oil and blend again. Serve garnished with fresh cilantro.

 Turmeric is related to ginger and when ground, looks similar, but this bitter yellow root is most commonly used as one of the ingredients in curry powder. Curcumin is the active ingredient in turmeric; it has high amounts of antioxidants, manganese, and iron, and is also an excellent anti-inflammatory.

SPICY MEXICAN LIME SOUP

MAKES 2–4 SERVINGS

Full of flavor and heat, this fiery soup will take the chill out of any day! If you don't like spicy food, you can omit the hot peppers, but I encourage you to add just a little. Serve with Guacamole (p. 131) and dehy-drated crackers for the perfect meal.

1 cup (250 mL) chopped tomatoes

¼ cup (60 mL) red onions

1 garlic clove

2 cups (500 mL) chopped, peeled cucumber

3 tbsp lime juice

1 tsp Himalayan salt

dash cayenne pepper

½–1 jalapeño or habañero pepper with seeds,
   to taste

1 avocado, chopped

1 tbsp extra virgin olive oil

1 cup (250 mL) chopped, packed fresh cilantro

2 tbsp chopped cilantro, for garnish

In a blender, process 1 cup (250 mL) purified water, tomatoes, onions, garlic, cucumber, lime juice, salt, cayenne pepper, and hot pepper until smooth. Add avocado, olive oil, and 1 cup cilantro, blending again. Season to taste. Garnish with 2 tbsp cilantro.

Capsaicin, the hot pepper's natural heat-causing component, has been used to improve heart health, prevent sinus infections, break up cold congestion, alleviate pain, and reduce blood clot damage. Contrary to popular belief, hot peppers don't cause stomach ulcers, but may help to spike metabolism and burn fat.

CREAMY ZUCCHINI BISQUE

MAKES 2–4 SERVINGS

A simple fuss-free soup that can be made in just minutes—the perfect choice when you want something light, creamy, and good for you.

3 cups (750 mL) peeled, chopped zucchini

1 celery stalk, roughly chopped

1 tbsp lemon juice

1 tbsp light miso paste

½ tsp Himalayan salt

1 tsp onion powder

¼ cup (60 mL) hemp seeds

½ avocado, chopped

dash cayenne pepper, to taste

1 tbsp hemp seeds, for garnish

In a blender, process 2 cups (500 mL) purified water with zucchini, celery, lemon juice, miso, salt, onion powder, and hemp seeds until creamy. Add avocado and blend again. Season to taste and sprinkle with 1 tbsp hemp seeds.

➤ *Zucchinis and cucumbers often have a mild or intense bitter taste due to compounds called cucurbitacins. Always taste zucchini before using—when bitter, it can cause gas, diarrhea, and stomach cramps.*

➤ *Himalayan crystal salt is an unrefined pink salt that contains many trace minerals. All salt contains sodium, which can contribute to high blood pressure, heart disease, and water retention. All white salts (including sea salts) are highly processed and devoid of any nutrients. If your salt is pure white, it is missing minerals. All truly natural salts have a sandy tint.*

ALKALINE MINERAL BROTH

MAKES ABOUT 2 QT (2 L)

This broth is an alkalizing drink that supplies vitamins and minerals to the body. I often drink this during extended fasts, as it is particularly rich in potassium and other minerals, and has a very grounding effect. Feel free to add whatever veggies you have in the refrigerator!

 A natural source of sodium and important minerals, celery is very alkaline and high in fiber. Traditionally, it's been used to lower blood pressure.

3 large organic potatoes, chopped

1 cup (250 mL) yams, chopped

1 cup (250 mL) beets, chopped

2 cups (500 mL) chopped broccoli

1 cup (250 mL) chopped mixed dark green vegetables
(e.g., chard, kale, collard greens, spinach, watercress)

1 cup (250 mL) chopped celery

1 cup (250 mL) chopped red or green cabbage

1 cup (250 mL) chopped onions

about ½ cup (125 mL) chopped cilantro

about ½ cup (125 mL) chopped parsley

All vegetables should be chopped into 1-in (2.5-cm) dice. In a large stainless steel pot on high, bring 8 cups (2 L) purified water with all ingredients to a boil. Reduce heat, cover pot, and simmer slowly for about 60 minutes. Remove from heat. Strain broth into a large glass jar or bowl. *Be careful when handling hot liquids!*

If you're not fasting, you can eat the cooked veggies. If not used immediately, keep broth in refrigerator. Warm before serving.

SOUP STOCK

MAKES ABOUT 7 CUPS (1.75 mL)

A good (cooked) soup starts with a good stock! Keep vegetable trimmings, leaves, and stems on hand to add to stock. Certain herbs, spices, and vegetables add a distinct taste to dishes, but this stock is "neutral," no one flavor dominates, and so it complements a variety of sauces, stews, and soups. It's also good to drink as a snack between meals and, when served with grains, dumplings, or legumes, becomes a complete meal.

1 large onion

2 small unpeeled potatoes

1 large carrot

½ cup (125 mL) roughly chopped yam

1 medium tomato

2 cups (500 mL) broccoli stems

1 cup (250 mL) chopped zucchini

6–8 fresh parsley sprigs with leaves

2–3 fresh thyme sprigs or 1 tsp dried thyme

4 bay leaves

7 whole black peppercorns

5 whole cloves

1 tsp dried lovage (or a few fresh sprigs)

3 large garlic cloves

1 tbsp + 1 tsp chopped fresh ginger

dash cayenne pepper

1 tsp dried basil (or a few fresh sprigs)

1 tsp dried chervil (or a few fresh sprigs)

Chop all vegetables into 1-in (2.5-cm) dice. In a large pot on medium, slowly bring 8 cups (2 L) purified water to a boil with all ingredients, except basil and chervil. Reduce heat, cover pot, and simmer gently for 50 minutes, stirring occasionally. (The longer the soup simmers, the richer the flavor.) Add basil and chervil in last 15 minutes. Remove from heat and allow stock to cool slightly. While still warm, strain through a fine sieve, pressing down hard with a spoon on the vegetables to squeeze out all the juices. *Be careful when handling hot liquids!* Discard vegetables and refrigerate or freeze stock.

WILD GARLIC (OR LEEK) SOUP

MAKES 2–4 SERVINGS

Wild garlic is harvested only in the spring and sold in little bunches at farmer's markets. It tastes similar to domestic garlic, but is slightly milder.

1 small carrot, roughly chopped

1 small onion, roughly chopped

1 small potato, roughly chopped

1 celery stalk, roughly chopped

½ bunch wild garlic bulbs and stems, about 1 cup (250 mL), or 2 cups (500 mL) sliced leeks and 3 large garlic cloves, grated

1 bay leaf

½ cup (125 mL) wild garlic, chopped (or 1 cup [250 mL] thinly sliced leeks)

1 medium carrot, sliced thinly

½ tsp dried basil

½ tsp dried thyme

½ tsp dried tarragon

⅛ tsp cayenne pepper

1 cup (250 mL) almond or nut-free mylk

½ cup (125 mL) minced fresh parsley

1 tsp Himalayan salt

In a large pot on high, bring to a boil 3 cups (750 mL) water, carrots, onions, potatoes, celery, ½ bunch wild garlic, sliced leeks and 3 garlic cloves, and bay leaf. Let simmer for about 20 minutes. Remove from heat. Remove bay leaf. Allow soup to cool. In a blender, purée until smooth.

While soup is cooling, in a small pot on medium, cook 1 cup (250 mL) water, ½ cup (125 mL) wild garlic, salt, and sliced carrots for about 15 minutes.

Return puréed soup to pot, and add cooked garlic, carrot, and water from small pot. Stir in basil, thyme, tarragon, cayenne, and mylk. Stirring soup well with wooden spoon, simmer gently for 5 minutes to reheat. Season to taste and garnish with parsley.

About Garlic

A clove of garlic a day keeps the doctor away! Garlic is a natural antibiotic, and has also been used to treat heart disease, immune disorders, candida, ear-aches, arthritis, and more. This super bulb is a strong antiseptic, lowers blood pressure and cholesterol, reduces blood clotting, and offers protection against cardiovascular illness. It strengthens the body's defences against colds, infections, and intestinal dis-orders. Applied to the skin, it keeps mosquitoes away. And when my mother suffered from a pulmonary embolism in her leg, she began to eat more garlic (up to 8 cloves a day!) to promote blood flow.

Garlic's healing powers have played an important role throughout history. Legend has it that the slaves who built the pyramids in Egypt were fed a daily diet of garlic to build up their strength. When the plague raged throughout Europe in the Middle Ages, it is said that those who ate garlic were spared from getting sick. And during World War I, Russian doctors treated infections and wounds with garlic (which is why it was called the Russian penicillin). For many centuries, it was believed that garlic could also ward off vampires.

In the kitchen, garlic enhances soups, salads, and many raw and cooked dishes. Before consuming garlic, press, grate, chop, or mince it and expose it to air for ten minutes.

To freshen your breath after eating garlic, chew a few fennel, caraway, or cardamom seeds or a sprig of chlorophyll-rich fresh parsley.

 "When I was growing up, garlic was believed to be a cure-all. Twice a year, I had to drink hot garlic milk at bedtime as a cure for pinworms. To treat colds and fevers, my mother strung garlic cloves on a twine. After two nights of having to sleep with this necklace, I was healthy and back in school!" —Ilse

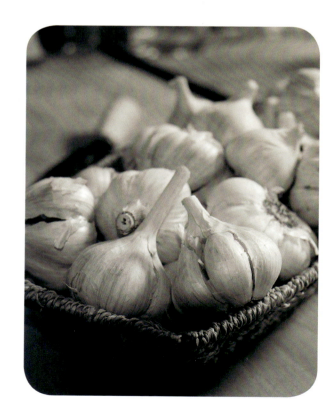

Soups

TOMATO-MILLET SOUP

MAKES 4–6 SERVINGS

I asked my mother to include the recipe for this
delicious soup—my childhood favorite—in our book. I
hope you enjoy it as much as I used to!

2 small potatoes, unpeeled, chopped into 1-in (2.5-cm)
   dice
1 cup (250 mL) coarsely chopped onions
1 cup (250 mL) coarsely chopped carrots
1 cup (250 mL) coarsely chopped fennel bulb
3 large tomatoes or 2 cups (500 mL) tomato juice
1 garlic clove, grated or pressed
1 bay leaf
1 tsp ground ginger
1 tsp ground dried rosemary leaves
½ tsp dried basil
½ tsp apple cider vinegar
1 tsp salt, or to taste
1 cup (250 mL) cooked millet
3–4 tbsp chopped fresh dill, for garnish

In a large pot on high, bring to a boil 4 cups (1 L) purified water or soup stock (p. 94) with potatoes, onions,
carrots, fennel, tomatoes, garlic, and bay leaf. Reduce
heat to medium and let simmer, covered, for about 20
minutes. Remove from heat. Remove bay leaf. When
soup is cool enough to handle, in a blender, purée
until smooth.

Return soup to pot, and add remainder of ingredients, except dill. Reheat on low and let simmer
for about 10 minutes. Season to taste. Serve with a
generous sprinkling of fresh dill.

BABUSCHKA'S BORSCHT

This was a staple in our Eastern European household, although my mother would include a beef bone in the soup, at my father's request. Babushka means grandmother in Russian; here is her veganized and much healthier version.

▶ *"Russian borscht is a hearty soup that makes a meal when served with dark rye bread. The flavor gets even better after a day or two, and the soup also tastes delicious when served cold on a hot summer day. Serve it with a bowl of Sour Kream (p. 132) on the side." —Ilse*

1 cup (250 mL) finely chopped onions

1 cup (250 mL) finely chopped tomatoes

1 large carrot, julienned

3 medium beets, julienned

2 bay leaves

2 tbsp ground dill seeds

2 medium potatoes, cubed

1 cup (250 mL) orange bell peppers, thinly sliced

1 cup (250 mL) string beans, thinly sliced

1 cup (250 mL) coarsely chopped green cabbage

3 garlic cloves, grated or pressed

1 tbsp dried marjoram

1 tbsp dried thyme

2 cups (500 mL) beet greens, if fresh, finely chopped (optional)

1 cup (250 mL) cooked kidney beans, optional

1 tsp Himalayan salt, or to taste

¼ cup (60 mL) lemon juice

¼ tsp red pepper flakes or cayenne pepper

½ cup (125 mL) chopped fresh dill

In a large pot on high, bring to a boil 8 cups (2 L) purified water with onions, tomatoes, carrots, beets, bay leaves, and dill seeds. Reduce heat and gently simmer for 30 minutes, stirring occasionally. Add potatoes, bell peppers, string beans, cabbage, garlic, marjoram, and thyme and cook for another 15 minutes, until vegetables are cooked but not mushy. Add beet greens and kidney beans, if using, and heat, but don't allow them to cook. Add salt, lemon juice, red pepper flakes or cayenne, and fresh dill. Season to taste.

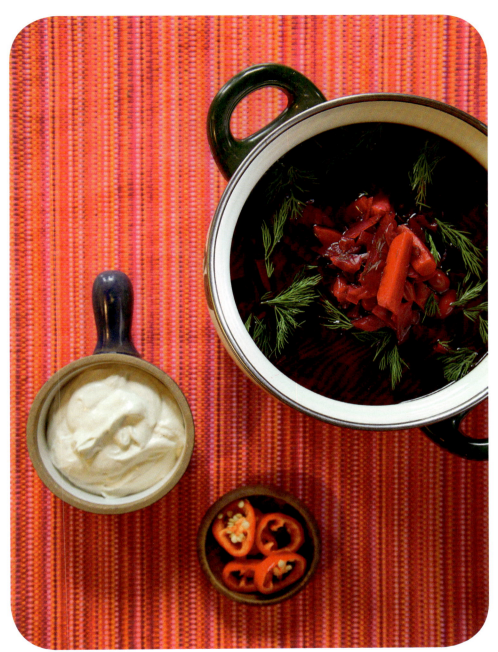

Dill is a favorite in Russian cooking. It is best used fresh, as cooking diminishes the flavor. The seeds are used to season soups and sauces, and in pickling sauerkraut and cucumbers. Medicinally, dill is good for indigestion. Dill water was given as a soothing drink to wailing infants and was said to promote milk in nursing mothers. There are also many ancient superstitions concerning dill; it was once believed to counteract spells cast by witches and sorcerers.

CAULIFLOWER CHOWDER

MAKES 4–5 SERVINGS

Thick, hearty, and delicious—the perfect remedy for a cold winter day! When my mother used to make this soup, I would always sneak a few cauliflower florets to eat raw. I hope you will too! **Note:** For a nut-free soup, use coconut mylk.

1 small head cauliflower

1 medium yam, coarsely chopped

1 medium onion, coarsely chopped

1 medium carrot, coarsely chopped

2 medium potatoes, coarsely chopped

1 celery stalk, coarsely chopped

1 bay leaf

1 tsp Himalayan salt

1 tsp dried basil

½ tsp ground or grated nutmeg

1 cup (250 mL) finely chopped parsley

1 cup (250 mL) almond or coconut mylk

freshly ground black pepper, to taste

Cut about 2 cups (500 mL) cauliflower into small florets and set aside. In a large pot on medium, cook remaining cauliflower (coarsely chopped), yam, onions, carrots, potatoes, celery, and bay leaf in 5 cups (1.25 mL) purified water or soup stock (p. 94) for about 20 minutes. Remove from heat. Remove bay leaf. In a blender, purée soup until creamy. *Be careful when blending hot liquids!*

Return blended liquid to pot, add cauliflower florets and salt, and cook on medium heat for another 10 minutes. Stir in basil, nutmeg, parsley, and mylk and allow to heat, about 5 minutes. Season to taste with additional salt, if desired, and black pepper.

LENTIL SOUP WITH KALE

MAKES 4–5 SERVINGS

When we celebrate New Year's Eve with my Mexican sister-in-law Maru, my family eats lentil soup at midnight followed by 12 grapes, each symbolizing a month of good luck for the coming year. The lentils dissolve while cooking and make the soup creamy.

1 cup (250 mL) red lentils, well rinsed

1 bay leaf

1 medium onion, finely chopped

1 large carrot, diced

1 celery stalk, diced

1 small yam, cubed

1 tsp dried marjoram

1 tsp ground cumin

1 tsp ground coriander seeds

1 tsp ground fennel seeds

2 cups (500 mL) finely chopped kale

2 garlic cloves garlic, pressed or grated

2 tsp salt, or to taste

⅛ tsp cayenne pepper, or to taste

1 cup cilantro, for garnish

In a large pot on high, bring to a boil 6 cups (1.5 mL) purified water, lentils, bay leaf, onions, carrots, celery, yam, marjoram, cumin, and coriander and fennel seeds. Skim off any foam from top of water. Cook partly covered for about 20 minutes, stirring occasionally. Add kale, garlic, and salt and simmer for another 10–15 minutes. Remove bay leaf, stir in cayenne, and serve garnished with fresh cilantro.

About Miso

According to Japanese folklore, miso was a gift from the gods to ensure health and long life. Although rich in enzymes and probiotics, miso isn't raw. It is used not only in soups, but also in vegetable dishes, dressings, pickles, and various condiments. Japanese studies show that miso regulates blood sugar and contains healthy live bacterial cultures, antioxidants, and minerals. Miso has an alkalizing effect on the body and strengthens the immune system. Whenever I feel a cold coming on, I prepare a quick broth using miso paste, hot water, cayenne, and tons of raw garlic to ward it off.

Miso is most often made from soybeans, but other varieties are made from rice, barley, and chickpeas. I prefer an unpasteurized, light, mild-tasting miso (shiro miso) and often use it as a seasoning in place of salt. It's not a pure raw food, but the fermentation process adds enzymes and beneficial bacteria. Make sure to look for miso that's organic and hasn't been genetically modified.

A note on soy: Soy products, such as veggie burgers, mock meat slices, and soy dogs, can be a good transition food when shifting away from a meat-based diet. However, they are highly processed and often contain unhealthy additives. Less processed soy foods—miso, tamari, tempeh, and edamame (soy beans)—are richer in nutrients and easier to digest. Always choose organic soy products; commercial soy is genetically modified.

MISO SOUP WITH SHIITAKE MUSHROOMS

MAKES 4 SERVINGS

Miso is a fermented soy product loaded with beneficial bacteria and enzymes. Use unpasteurized rice or chickpea miso for a gluten-free soup.

1 cup (250 mL) julienned carrots

1 cup (250 mL) julienned turnips

1 cup (250 mL) thinly sliced celery

1 cup (250 mL) thinly sliced onions

4 shiitake mushrooms, soaked for 10 minutes and
    thinly sliced, stems discarded

2 tbsp grated fresh ginger

3 tbsp miso, or to taste

½ cup (125 mL) sliced scallions or watercress, for
    garnish

In a large pot on high, bring to a boil 5 cups (1.25 L) purified water with all ingredients, except ginger, miso, and scallions. Reduce heat to medium-low and cook for 20 minutes. Add ginger after about 15 minutes. In a small bowl, combine miso with a few tbsp of hot broth; mix into a smooth paste, and return to soup. Do not let it boil again. Serve garnished with scallions or watercress.

Shiitake mushrooms are nutritious and beneficial for the immune system. They are a rich source of iron, zinc, B vitamins (especially niacin and riboflavin,) magnesium, potassium, selenium, and amino acids.

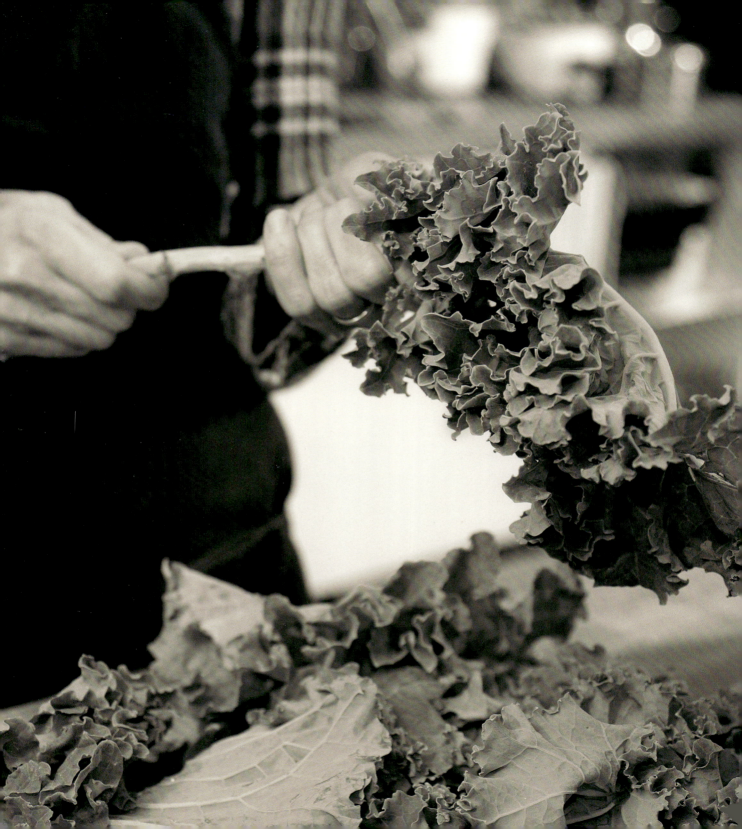

SALADS & SALAD DRESSINGS

Crispy Romaine & Beets with Garlic Dressing 107

Baby Greens with Sweet Miso Dressing 108

Garden Salad with Creamy Tahini Dressing 109

The Mason Jar Salad 110

Garden Salad in a Jar 111

Over-the-Top Taco Salad in a Jar 112

About Kale 113

Super Natural Kale 114

Bombay Kale 115

Award-Winning Marinated Kale Salad 116

Potluck Surprise Slaw 117

Wild about Rice Salad 118

Spicy Thai Salad 120

Kyssa House Dressing 122

Basil Balsamic Dressing 122

Creamy Peppercorn Dressing 123

Sweet Mustard Dressing 123

Avocado Dill Dressing 124

Frugal Rice Salad 124

Dandelion Potato Salad 125

Austrian Blauekraut 126

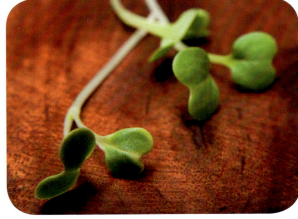

Most of the time, salad is treated like the least important part of a meal and served as an appetizer or side dish. But salads are a terrific source of valuable live nutrients that are not always available from the cooked "main course." For many raw foodists, like me, salads are the main event. They provide vitamins, minerals, enzymes, and important phytonutrients that can help protect against diseases and maximize health. Pound for pound, leafy greens supply more vitamins than red meat. They also contain enzymes to help break down food during digestion, providing more energy with less digestive effort.

Long before I became a raw foodist, I loved salads, thanks to my mother, who really knew how to dress them up. They were my favorite part of the meal—I frequently had second and even third helpings, and ate directly from the serving bowl when (I thought) no one was looking. Today, I prefer to eat my salad in a nicely shaped wooden bowl with chopsticks, to ensure that I eat slowly.

Salads are incredibly simple to prepare—all you need is a decent knife, chopping board, and salad bowl. They can be created from almost any vegetable and offer a multitude of colors, textures, and flavors. They can be made more substantial by adding a scoop of pâté or topped with extra ingredients such as organic raisins, goji berries, nuts, seeds, or avocados. For me, a salad isn't complete without sprouts or micro-greens. I used to add a lightly steamed yam or baked potato drizzled with flax oil to my salads to make them more filling; you can also try steamed broccoli, asparagus, green beans, or even quinoa. With quality, seasonal ingredients, an ordinary salad can be made into an extraordinary meal.

About Oils

Most oils have a limited shelf life and go rancid quickly as they age and are exposed to air and light. Purchase olive, nut, and seed oils in well-sealed dark glass bottles and store in a cool, dry place, away from direct light and heat. Store flax and hemp oils in the refrigerator. Before using oil, make sure it doesn't smell rancid. Use within three months to ensure that the healthy phytonutrients remain intact.

When making salad dressings, you can use less oil if you partially or completely replace it with water. A piece of avocado is a great alternative to oil in many dressings and sauces.

About Vinegars

Raw, unfiltered, and unpasteurized apple cider vinegar is the only form of vinegar that is alkaline-forming. Made from fermented apples, apple cider vinegar is naturally rich in beneficial enzymes. It is recommended to soothe sore throats and digestive upsets, treat acne, and more.

White vinegar is extremely acidic and I don't think it's fit for consumption; however, it's great for cleaning kitchen counters, cutting boards, stainless steel appliances, windows, and sinks!

Richly flavored balsamic vinegar isn't raw (it's boiled-down and fermented wine vinegar), but some raw foodists use it sparingly.

CRISPY ROMAINE & BEETS WITH GARLIC DRESSING

MAKES 4 SERVINGS

Garlic, beets, and raisins makes this iron-rich salad burst with color and flavor. It makes a delicious winter meal.

> *Beets are an excellent source of easily absorbed plant iron, which helps build healthy blood. Thanks to their betalain, which gives them their red pigment, beets are considered an anti-cancer food. They are also rich in potassium, calcium, phosphorous, folate, and vitamins A and C. Beets have been used traditionally to support healthy liver function and help cure liver ailments.*

1 head chopped romaine lettuce

1 cup (250 mL) diced beets

1 cup (250 mL) chopped cauliflower

½ cup (125 mL) Thompson raisins

2 green onions, thinly sliced

Garlic Dressing:

¼ cup (60 mL) extra virgin olive oil

¼ cup (60 mL) lemon juice

2 garlic cloves, pressed or grated

3 tbsp gluten-free tamari

2 tbsp maple syrup or 2–3 drops stevia extract

½ tsp dried tarragon

In a large bowl, combine all salad ingredients. In a jar, combine dressing ingredients. Seal jar and shake well. Toss dressing with salad. Dressing will keep 1 week in the refrigerator.

BABY GREENS WITH SWEET MISO DRESSING

MAKES 2–4 SERVINGS;
MAKES ABOUT 1 CUP (250 mL) DRESSING

Micro-greens (edible, tender greens produced from vegetables, herbs, or other plants) are harvested when very young, tiny, and full of live nutrients. They can be grown at home or purchased from a local grower. The delicate balance of miso, sesame, and ginger in the dressing gives this salad an Asian touch; keep some in the refrigerator to use with any salad.

4 cups mixed baby greens (romaine, spinach, etc.)
2 cups (500 mL) micro-greens
6 radishes, finely sliced
½ English cucumber, thinly sliced
3 tbsp black sesame seeds, for garnish

Sweet Miso Dressing:

½ cup (125 mL) purified water, or more, to taste
½ cup (125 mL) raw tahini
3 tbsp light miso
1 tbsp + 1 tsp chopped fresh ginger
3 tbsp maple syrup or 2–3 drops stevia
1 tbsp tamari
1 tbsp toasted sesame oil (optional)

In a large salad bowl, combine all salad ingredients except sesame seeds and set aside. In a blender, process all dressing ingredients until smooth. Toss salad with dressing just before serving. Garnish with black sesame seeds.

GARDEN SALAD WITH CREAMY TAHINI DRESSING

MAKES 2–4 SERVINGS

Here's a perfectly balanced, rich, and tangy dressing that's especially delicious on romaine leaves. It can also be enjoyed as a dip served with vegetables of your choice. Make it in advance and keep it in the refrigerator—but it tastes so good, it won't last very long!

1 head romaine lettuce, torn into bite-sized pieces
½ English cucumber, thinly sliced
1 cup (250 mL) halved cherry tomatoes
1 cup (250 mL) sliced orange bell peppers
about ½ cup (125 mL) sunflower sprouts, for garnish

Creamy Tahini Dressing:

⅓ cup (80 mL) purified water (adjust for thickness)
2 cloves garlic
2 tbsp gluten-free tamari
1 tbsp lemon juice
2 tbsp apple cider vinegar
¼ cup (60 mL) raw tahini
dash cayenne pepper (optional)
¼ cup (60 mL) extra virgin olive oil

In a large salad bowl, combine all salad ingredients except sprouts. In a blender, process water, garlic, tamari, lemon juice, and vinegar until garlic is thoroughly blended. Add tahini, cayenne, and oil, and blend again. Season to taste. Toss salad with dressing just before serving. Garnish with sprouts.

The Mason Jar Salad

The reliable old-fashioned Mason jar is truly indispensable for summer jams and jellies as well as pickled autumn vegetables, for soaking and sprouting nuts, seeds, and legumes, and for drinking ever-popular green concoctions from. It also has become the latest trend in on-the-go healthy eating.

The Mason jar salad is a fresh alternative to those stored in standard Tupperware. The easy-to-transport (and clean) glass jar showcases the vibrant colors of the layered ingredients—guaranteed to impress your co-workers!

The fun thing about these beautiful salads is that you can get creative and experiment with different vegetables and dressings. I usually layer the heaviest items on the bottom, but really there are no set rules—as long as you start with the dressing or sauce and end with the more delicate lettuces and sprouts on top. Layered salads can be prepared up to three days in advance, and they will stay fresh in the refrigerator as long as the dressing at the bottom of the jar does not touch the greens until you're ready to eat it. This is the most important principle.

Use a variety of whichever dressings, greens, vegetables, and colorful toppings you enjoy. Make a bunch of these little beauties on Sunday so they're waiting for you in the refrigerator during the work week. A quart-sized jar makes one big, meal-sized salad. Divide between two people or enjoy as a main course like I do.

Note: This is a fun kitchen project in which to involve your children!

- First, pour salad dressing into a wide-mouthed Mason jar.
- Layer heartier vegetables and those that need to marinate on the bottom of the jar, starting with wetter ingredients (such as shredded cabbage, julienned carrots, chickpeas, lentils, black beans, radish, onions, cauliflower, broccoli, kale, sweet potatoes, and mushrooms).
- Next, add a layer of softer vegetables (such as cucumbers, corn, tomatoes, peas, zucchini, or avocado sprinkled with lemon juice to prevent browning).
- Tempeh, gluten-free grains, lentils, and pastas are nice add-ons. If you're using them, place them toward the top of the jar so they don't get soggy in the dressing.
- Add nuts, seeds, and dried fruits.
- Place the lightest ingredients—delicate greens that you don't want touching the dressing—at the top of the jar, or they'll become soggy.
- Top with fresh and colorful herbs, sprouts, micro-greens, or edible flowers.
- Leave a little headspace at the top of the jar so that you have enough room to toss the salad.
- Fasten lid tightly.

- When you're ready to eat, turn the jar upside down and shake to coat all the layers of vegetables. You can also transfer the salad into a bowl and toss, but it's more fun to eat directly from the jar!

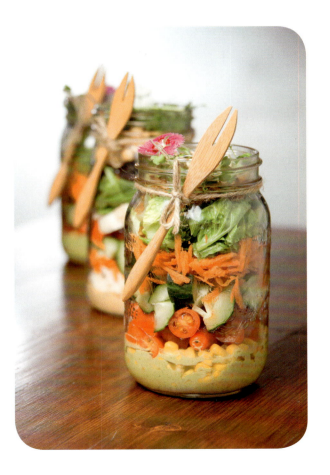

GARDEN SALAD IN A JAR

MAKES 2–4 SERVINGS

A vibrant presentation that transforms a simple salad into something special! If you don't have all the ingredients, just use the ones you have.

6 tbsp dressing of choice (see pp. 122–124)
1 cup (125 mL) chopped cauliflower
½ cup (125 mL) shredded carrots
1 cup (125 mL) sliced radishes
1 cup (125 mL) sliced mushrooms
¾ cup (125 mL) chickpeas, sprouted or cooked
½ cup (125 mL) halved grape tomatoes
2 cups (500 mL) baby spinach leaves
½ cup (125 mL) Thompson raisins
about ½ cup (125 mL) micro-greens
edible flowers, for garnish

Divide above ingredients between 2 1-qt/L Mason Jars, beginning with 3 tbsp of salad dressing in bottom of each jar. Add remainder of ingredients in order listed, one layer at a time.

OVER-THE-TOP TACO SALAD IN A JAR

MAKES 2–4 SERVINGS;

DRESSING MAKES ABOUT ¾ CUP (185 mL)

A fabulous new way to enjoy an old standby! This is
also delicious with a layer of Pico De Gallo salsa
(p. 131).

6 tbsp Cilantro Lime Dressing

1 cup (250 mL) corn, fresh or frozen and thawed

½ cup (125 mL) halved grape tomatoes

½ cup (125 mL) diced cucumbers

½ cup (125 mL) diced orange bell peppers

2 tbsp finely chopped green or red onions

½ avocado, diced

2 cups (500 mL) chopped romaine lettuce

½ cup (125 mL) walnut "Neat" (p. 162)

½ cup (125 mL) micro-greens and/or sprouts

2 tbsp minced cilantro

edible flowers, for garnish

Cilantro Lime Dressing:

1 cup (125 mL) minced cilantro

1 tbsp hemp seeds

¼ cup (60 mL) extra virgin olive oil

¼ cup (60 mL) lime juice

1 small garlic clove, chopped (optional)

2 tsp maple syrup

½ tsp Himalayan salt

½-in–2-in (1–5-cm) slice jalapeño pepper (optional)

dash freshly ground black pepper, to taste

In a blender, process all dressing ingredients until
smooth. Season to taste. Divide ingredients between
2 1-qt/L Mason jars, beginning with 3 tbsp dressing.
Layer remainder of ingredients in order, one at a time,
saving sprouts and edible flowers for last.

About Kale

Kale is a nutritional powerhouse packed with amino acids, vitamins A, B, C, and K, and important phytochemicals that help protect against disease. It also contains impressive amounts of calcium, potassium, magnesium, and iron necessary for strong bones and beautiful skin.

Although highly nutritious, raw kale and other cruciferous vegetables can be difficult to digest raw because of their tough outer cell walls (cellulose). Massaging the leaves breaks down the cellulose and wilts the kale, making it easier to digest.

Kale needs thorough washing too, as the leaves and stems are likely to have sand or dirt or even bugs clinging to them. Fill a sink or large bowl with water and submerge kale in it, swishing it around and allowing the grit to settle; repeat if necessary. After washing, remove stems from leaves. Reserve stems for green juice or soup broths. To cut, stack leaves on top of one another, roll into tight bundles, and slice thinly (the technique is called chiffonade). Massage the leaves for a few minutes with a pinch of salt and about 1 tbsp lemon juice. This results in soft and tender kale, as if steamed, but much more nutritious.

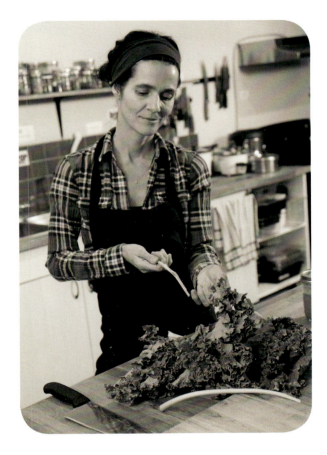

SUPER NATURAL KALE

MAKES 2–4 SERVINGS

Addictively delicious, delightfully nutritious—this salad
is bound to be a favorite for all who experience it!

1 large head curly kale, stems removed and leaves
   chopped finely

1 small orange bell pepper, seeded and diced

¼ tsp Himalayan salt

½ cup chopped sundried tomatoes

¼ cup (60 mL) soaked goji berries

¼ cup (60 mL) mung bean sprouts

3–4 tbsp apple cider vinegar

3 tbsp extra virgin olive oil

1–2 tsp maple syrup

1 tbsp gluten-free tamari

dash cayenne pepper, to taste

1 large garlic clove, grated or pressed

1 avocado, diced

¼ cup (60 mL) sauerkraut (optional)

Soak sundried tomatoes in 1 cup water for 30 minutes.
Drain and rinse.

In a large mixing bowl, massage kale leaves with
salt until kale softens. (Keep at it, you're nearly there!)
Add remainder of ingredients, except for sauerkraut,
and toss to combine well. Season to taste. Serve
topped with sauerkraut for an extra immunity boost!

➤ *Sauerkraut is a dietary staple in Austria and has
many uses in folk medicine. Father Sebastian
Kneipp, a nineteenth-century Austrian herbalist
and healer, described sauerkraut as a "broom
which sweeps death and sickness out of the
intestines." Sauerkraut (along with wheatgrass,
sprouts, and Energy Soup) is a major component
of Dr Ann Wigmore's Living Foods Lifestyle
program (**annwigmore.org**), which has been
used by many people to overcome serious
illnesses. It helps fight against disease caused
by bacteria and has high amounts of enzymes,
natural probiotics, and vitamins. Sauerkraut
eaters are believed to live long, healthy lives. Eat
sauerkraut raw; cooking destroys its beneficial
effects.*

BOMBAY KALE

MAKES 4–6 SERVINGS

This salad has always impressed people when I've prepared it at festivals, shows, and dinners over the years. It has an exotic Indian flavor and is guaranteed to get reluctant kale eaters hooked on the mighty green. It is outrageously delicious!

2 heads green kale, finely chopped
1 orange bell pepper, seeded and diced
½ cup (125 mL) cherry tomatoes
¼ cup (60 mL) pumpkin seeds, for garnish (optional)
¼ cup (60 mL) Thompson raisins, for garnish (optional)
¼ cup (60 mL) sprouts or micro-greens, for garnish

Dressing:
¼ cup (60 mL) purified water
2 tsp chopped fresh ginger
4 garlic cloves, pressed or grated
¼ cup (60 mL) fresh lemon juice
¼ cup (60 mL) gluten-free tamari
4 pitted Medjool dates
2 tbsp curry powder
dash cayenne pepper
¼ cup (60 mL) extra virgin olive oil

In a large bowl, combine salad ingredients, except garnishes, and set aside. In a blender, process all dressing ingredients until smooth, adding more water if needed. Keep refrigerated until ready to use. If the dressing becomes too thick, add a bit more water. Pour as much dressing as you want over the kale and allow to marinate for 2 hours. If you wish to speed things along, use your hands to massage kale. Once softened, kale will shrink. Add garnishes before serving.

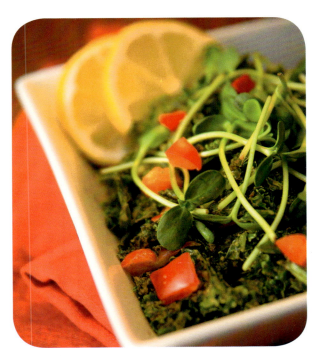

AWARD-WINNING MARINATED KALE SALAD

MAKES 2–4 SERVINGS

Awarded the *Ottawa Citizen* Readers' Favorite Recipe of 2007 by Ron Eade, former food editor at the *Citizen*—and carnivore. After tasting this salad, he wrote that he was inspired to pick up a few heads of kale to massage when he returned home! Serve this salad as a side or—as we do—a main dish.

1 large head kale, stems removed, and leaves finely chopped
½ tsp Himalayan salt
2 tbsp lemon juice
1 orange or yellow bell pepper, seeded and chopped
½ cup (125 mL) halved cherry tomatoes

Dressing:

1 garlic clove
1 celery stalk, roughly chopped
2 tbsp lemon juice
¼ cup (60 mL) extra virgin olive oil
1 tsp gluten-free tamari
1 avocado, chopped
dash cayenne pepper (optional)

In a large bowl, sprinkle salt over kale, then massage with your hands until the kale wilts, about 3–5 minutes. Add lemon juice and massage again for about 1 minute. Add bell peppers and tomatoes and toss.

In a blender, purée all dressing ingredients until creamy. Pour over kale and toss to combine well.

POTLUCK SURPRISE SLAW

MAKES 4–6 SERVINGS

Since 2006, my husband Mark and I have been organizing raw vegan potlucks in Ottawa as a fun way to bring our community together and to experience healthy eating. The events have been a great success over the years; the largest was attended by more than 150 people who brought an incredible variety of beautiful, lovingly prepared raw-food dishes. My mother has been an integral part of the potlucks since the beginning and often brings this Surprise Slaw.

1 cup (250 mL) red cabbage, roughly shredded with
   a grater
3 cups (750 mL) tightly packed sauerkraut
1 small onion, finely chopped
1 small apple, cored and coarsely grated or chopped
5 juniper berries, coarsely crushed (in a coffee grinder
   or with a mortar and pestle)
1 tsp crushed caraway seeds
⅓ cup (80 mL) pumpkin seed oil
¼ cup (60 mL) sauerkraut juice
dash cayenne pepper
1 apple, thinly sliced, for garnish
½ cup (125 mL) pumpkin seeds, for garnish

In a large bowl, combine all ingredients except garnishes, and toss to combine. Garnish with apple slices and pumpkin seeds.

I first tasted pumpkin seed oil while visiting my grandmother in Austria in 2004. We ate it at almost every meal, drizzled over fresh sauerkraut purchased from a local farmer. I recently rediscovered pumpkin seed oil and enjoy it drizzled over a mix of sauerkraut, avocadoes, and micro-greens.

*"Pumpkin seed oil (**Kürbiskern öl**) was extensively used in the area of Austria where I was raised. It has a dark green color and is often referred to as 'green gold.' We used to dry pumpkin seeds in the sun, then brought them to the mill, where they were pressed into oil. We dipped plain dark rye bread into a mixture of grated garlic, chopped onions, and pumpkin seed oil." —Ilse*

WILD ABOUT RICE SALAD

This dish has a chewy, nutty flavor that is perfect to serve during autumn—or any season—for a filling meal or side dish. Feel free to get creative and add other ingredients.

MAKES 4–6 SERVINGS

2½ cups (625 mL) wild rice

1 cup (250 mL) diced yams

1 red bell pepper, seeded and chopped

2 green onions, minced

½ cup (125 mL) Thompson raisins

3 tbsp apple cider vinegar

¼ cup (60 mL) extra virgin olive oil

2 tbsp gluten-free tamari

1 tbsp maple syrup or 2–3 drops stevia (optional)

dash cayenne pepper

dash freshly ground black pepper

In a large bowl, submerge rice in at least double amount of filtered water. Let soak for 2 days; change water twice daily. When ready, rice will split open and become soft.

Rinse rice in fresh water and drain in a colander while prepping other ingredients. Transfer to a large bowl and add remainder of ingredients. Season to taste.

> *Wild rice is the seed of a tall aquatic grass indigenous to Canada and the northern US. It is high in protein, B vitamins, potassium, iron, calcium, and phosphorus. Although today some "wild rice" is still harvested wild, most is grown commercially from hybridized seeds.*

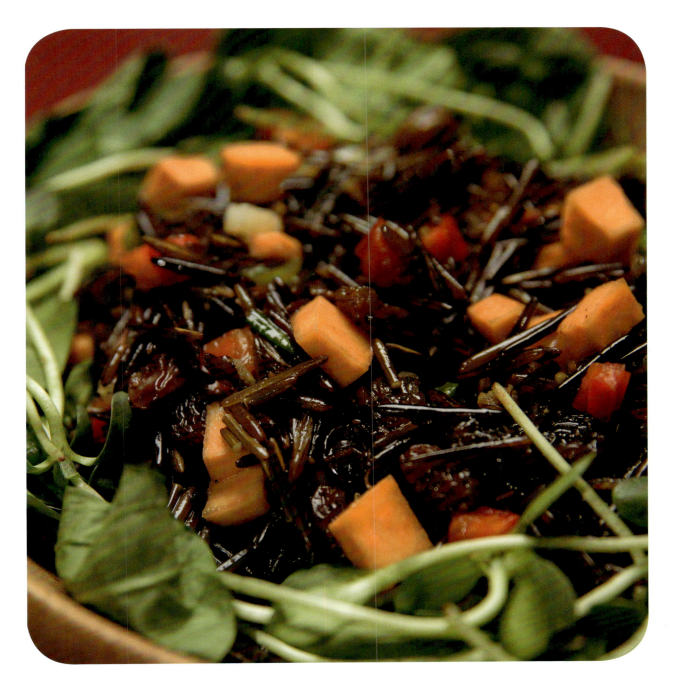

SPICY THAI SALAD

A wonderful, filling salad paired with a creamy dressing that has a hint of sesame. This will complement any meal.

MAKES 6 SERVINGS

6 cups (1.5 L) finely sliced green cabbage

1 cup (250 mL) finely sliced red cabbage

¼ cup (60 mL) finely chopped cilantro

1 large red bell pepper, seeded and diced

3 tbsp roughly chopped dry cashews, for garnish

Dressing:

½ cup (125 mL) raw sesame oil

2 tsp toasted sesame oil

¾ cup (185 mL) raw cashews, soaked for 30 minutes

¼ cup (60 mL) lime juice

3 tbsp gluten-free tamari

2 tbsp maple syrup

1–3 Thai chili peppers, to taste

¼ tsp Himalayan salt

1 heaping tbsp Irish Moss (optional)

In a large bowl, combine all salad ingredients and set aside. In a blender, purée all dressing ingredients until creamy. Season to taste. Pour dressing over salad and toss until well combined. The dressing will keep for up to 1 week in the refrigerator.

▶ *Also known as carrageenan, Irish moss is a sea vegetable used as a thickener. Once soaked and blended, Irish moss gives a fluffy texture to desserts. It can be used in recipes to reduce and partially replace fatty nuts and seeds.*

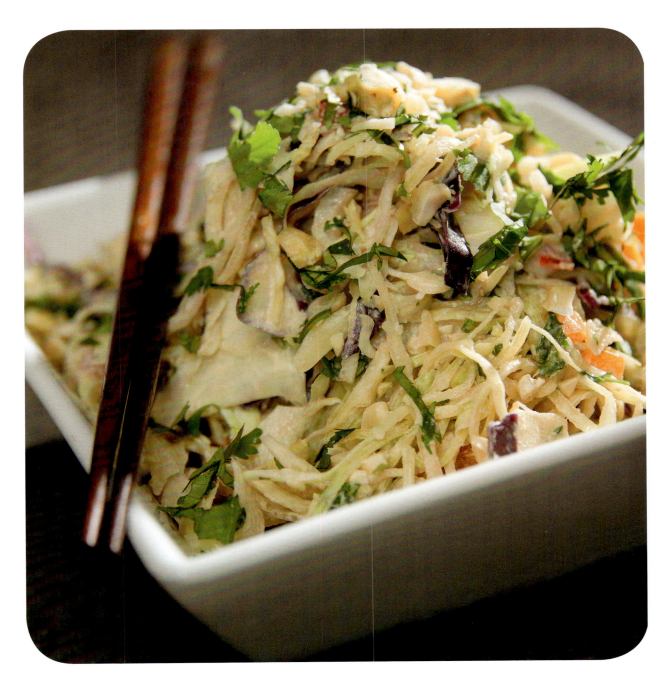

KYSSA HOUSE DRESSING

MAKES ABOUT ¾ CUP (185 mL)

A good salad dressing can make the difference between a boring bowl of lettuce and a meal that sings! This dressing is delicious with all greens. I've been making it for 20 years, and my family still asks for it. It will be a new favorite for your family, too!

¼ cup (60 mL) apple cider vinegar
½ cup (125 mL) flax seed oil
1 tbsp maple syrup
2 tbsp gluten-free tamari
1–3 garlic cloves, grated or pressed, to taste
dash cayenne pepper

In a glass jar with a lid, combine all ingredients. Seal jar and shake to combine well. Keeps for up to 5 days in the refrigerator.

➤ *When making salad dressings, you can use less oil if you partially or completely replace it with water. A piece of avocado is a great alternative to oil in many dressings and sauces.*

BASIL BALSAMIC DRESSING

MAKES ABOUT 1 CUP (250 mL)

A simple dressing that's great to have on hand in the refrigerator for up to 5 days. It is delicious on all mixed greens.

⅓ cup (80 mL) balsamic vinegar
⅔ cup (160 mL) extra virgin olive oil
1 tsp Dijon mustard
2 tsp finely minced fresh basil
1 tbsp gluten-free tamari
1 tsp maple syrup

In a jar with a lid, combine all ingredients. Seal jar and shake to combine well. Season to taste; if it is too sharp, add a little more oil.

➤ *"A pot of fresh sweet basil was always placed at the window of my mother's house to dispel flies, who avoid contact with the herb's pungent scent."*
—Ilse

CREAMY PEPPERCORN DRESSING

MAKES ABOUT 1 CUP (250 mL)

This creamy, omega-rich dressing will enhance any salad. It also makes a great dip for fresh garden vegetables. Watch out—it's addictive!

¼–½ cup (60–125 mL) purified water

½ cup (125 mL) hemp seeds

2 tbsp lemon juice

2 tbsp apple cider vinegar

2 tbsp gluten-free tamari

1 tbsp whole peppercorns

3 garlic cloves

1 tsp maple syrup or raw honey or 2–3 drops stevia extract

¾ cup (185 mL) extra virgin olive oil

In a blender, blend all ingredients except oil until creamy. Add oil and blend again. This dressing will keep for up to 5 days in the refrigerator.

SWEET MUSTARD DRESSING

MAKES ABOUT ¾ CUP (185 mL)

Honey-mustard dressing used to be one of my favorites; now I make it without the honey, and it's even better. Enjoy this sweet dressing on mixed greens or as a dip for sliced vegetables.

¼ cup (60 mL) apple cider vinegar

1 garlic clove, grated or pressed

3 tbsp maple syrup or other liquid sweetener or 2–3 drops stevia extract

3 tbsp prepared mustard

½ tsp Himalayan salt

¼ tsp freshly ground black pepper

½ cup (125 mL) extra virgin olive oil

In a jar, combine all ingredients and stir to combine. Seal jar and shake until silky smooth. Will keep for up to 1 week in refrigerator.

AVOCADO DILL DRESSING

MAKES ABOUT 1½ CUPS (375 mL)

An oil-free dressing that's both easy to make and delicious!

1 avocado, chopped
½–1 cup (125–250 mL) water, to taste
2½ tbsp lemon juice
¼ cup (60 mL) minced fresh dill
1 tsp gluten-free tamari
dash cayenne pepper, to taste
freshly ground black pepper, to taste

In a blender, purée all ingredients until creamy.

 Avocados are an excellent source of plant protein, potassium, magnesium, vitamins C, E, and K, and healthy, monounsaturated fats.

FRUGAL RICE SALAD

MAKES 6–7 SERVINGS

This salad makes a satisfying meal all on its own. For an attractive presentation, garnish with red pepper slices, black olives, and sunflower sprouts.

4 cups (1 L) cooked basmati rice
1 cup (250 mL) cooked black beans
1 cup (250 mL) chopped celery stalks and leaves
1 large carrot, coarsely grated
1 medium red onion, minced
½ cup (125 mL) finely chopped parsley
2 tsp dried thyme
1 tsp dried basil
1 tbsp ground coriander
2 tsp ground cumin
1 tbsp ground turmeric
2 tsp Himalayan salt
½ cup (125 mL) extra virgin olive oil
⅓ cup (80 mL) apple cider vinegar
¼ tsp cayenne pepper, or to taste

In a large bowl, toss all ingredients to combine well.

DANDELION & POTATO SALAD

MAKES 6 SERVINGS

This salad is popular in the region of Austria where my mother was born. It was one of her favorite meals in springtime when dandelions were in season.

Note: *If you're harvesting wild plants, make sure they haven't been sprayed with pesticides or grown near a busy road, where they will have absorbed toxic emissions.*

about 8 cups (2 L) chopped fresh dandelion leaves

2 large cooked potatoes, sliced

2 large garlic cloves, grated

1 tsp Himalayan salt

1 tsp dried basil

1 tsp crushed caraway or coriander seeds

⅓ cup (80 mL) pumpkin seed oil

¼ cup (60 mL) balsamic vinegar

In a large bowl, toss dandelion leaves with warm potatoes and remainder of ingredients until well combined.

*"The French call this herb **pis-en-lit** (wet-a-bed), which refers to its strong diuretic effect. Tea from the dandelion is said to be a blood purifier, stimulate the liver and gallbladder, and ease the pain of stiff joints. Dandelions have high levels of vitamins A, B, and C and iron. In folk medicine, it's believed that the sap from the stem fades age spots and, when repeatedly applied, removes warts. If you blow the white, fluffy seeds into the wind, it's believed that they will carry your thoughts to your loved one. Dried dandelion roots can be ground and roasted to make a delicious coffee substitute. A popular country wine is made from the leaves and flowers, and honey from the dandelion is beneficial to the liver." —Ilse*

AUSTRIAN BLAUKRAUT

MAKES 2–3 SERVINGS

Blaukraut is a traditional Austrian side dish, and it's a favorite at our family's Christmas meal. I used to make big batches and live on it for days at a time! Cooked cabbage in any form tastes even better when reheated the next day.

1 medium onion, finely chopped

3 cups (750 mL) sliced red cabbage

2 apples, cored and sliced

1 tsp caraway seeds

2 juniper berries, crushed

1 bay leaf

½ tsp ground cloves

½ tsp ground allspice

2 tbsp extra virgin olive oil

1 tsp Himalayan salt, or to taste

1 tbsp maple syrup

4 roasted chestnuts, quartered (optional)

2 tbsp apple cider vinegar or ½ cup (125 mL) dry red wine

In a large saucepan on medium heat, braise onions in ½ cup (125 mL) water for about 5 minutes. Add cabbage, apples, and another ½ cup water and cook for another 5 minutes, stirring constantly. Add remainder of ingredients except vinegar.

Partially cover saucepan, reduce heat to low, and cook for about 30 minutes, stirring frequently. Add more water if needed to prevent burning. Remove from heat, add vinegar, and remove bay leaf before serving.

 Chestnuts are low in calories and have high levels of vitamins B6 and C. They are a good source of magnesium, iron, and fiber. They have been traditionally used as a remedy for bronchitis, whooping cough, and irritations of the bronchial passages. My mother roasts chestnuts in a cast iron pan, while I eat them raw; they're equally delicious either way.

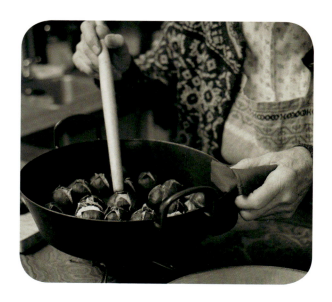

PÂTÉS, DIPS, SPREADS & CHEEZES

TuNO Pâté 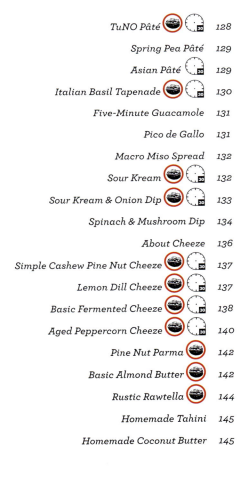 128

Spring Pea Pâté 129

Asian Pâté 129

Italian Basil Tapenade 130

Five-Minute Guacamole 131

Pico de Gallo 131

Macro Miso Spread 132

Sour Kream 132

Sour Kream & Onion Dip 133

Spinach & Mushroom Dip 134

About Cheeze 136

Simple Cashew Pine Nut Cheeze 137

Lemon Dill Cheeze 137

Basic Fermented Cheeze 138

Aged Peppercorn Cheeze 140

Pine Nut Parma 142

Basic Almond Butter 142

Rustic Rawtella 144

Homemade Tahini 145

Homemade Coconut Butter 145

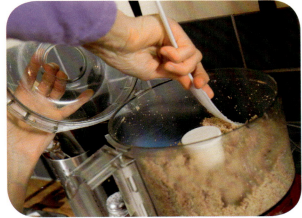

Rich and creamy, pâtés, dips, spreads, and cheezes are also versatile (try experimenting with different herbs and spices) and can transform a simple lunch into a tasty, satisfying meal. Pâtés can be enjoyed as a dip, a spread on cucumber rounds, or used to fill "sushi" or collard wraps. Most of these recipes can be prepared ahead of time and stored in the refrigerator.

When my mother ran her vegetarian tea room, The Pantry, in the 1970s, she was known for her unique vegetarian sandwich spreads and dips: Veggie pâté, tofu, mock "egg" salad, and The Pantry's famous cream cheese and cucumber spread were popular menu items. I continue to enjoy my own raw versions of many of her recipes, which are now appreciated by our customers at SimplyRaw Express.

tu**NO** PÂTÉ

MAKES ABOUT 5 CUPS (1 L)

I used to love tuna fish, and often heaped my mother's creamy, mayo-laden tuna on top of salads. Since becoming vegan, I've relied on this new favorite. Not only is it cholesterol-free, it's tuna- and dolphin-free—and it's also much tastier than the fishy stuff, whether served as a dip, a tasty salad topper, or stuffed in bell peppers or romaine leaves. If serving in wraps, top with sliced tomatoes, sprouts, green onions, and diced red cabbage.

1 garlic clove

¼ medium red onion, chopped

4 celery stalks, chopped

2 apples, cored and grated

2 cups (500 mL) walnuts, soaked for 8 hours

¼ cup (60 mL) apple cider vinegar

¼ cup (60 mL) gluten-free tamari

¼ cup (60 mL) extra virgin olive oil

1 tbsp dulse powder

½ tsp freshly ground black pepper

1 tsp dried basil

3 green onions, thinly sliced

1 medium carrot, grated

2–3 sprigs parsley, for garnish

In a food processor, blend garlic and onions. Add celery and process again. Add apples and process again. Add walnuts, vinegar, tamari, olive oil, dulse, black pepper, and basil, and process until smooth. Transfer to a large mixing bowl and stir in green onions and carrots. Season to taste. Garnish with parsley.

A red sea vegetable, dulse is an excellent source of minerals, trace elements, and organic iodine—an important nutrient for thyroid support. It comes in whole leaf or dried flake form, great for adding some saltiness to a recipe. Because it comes from the sea, dulse gives this recipe its fishy flavor.

SPRING PEA PÂTÉ

ASIAN PÂTÉ

MAKES ABOUT 3½ CUPS (830 mL)

Unlike most popular pâtés, which tend to be high in fat, this zesty crowd pleaser is low-fat yet incredibly flavorful. Serve with a platter of vegetables and crackers or spread on sliced zucchini and carrots for a colorful party presentation.

2 garlic cloves
4 cups fresh or frozen (and thawed) peas
juice of 2 large limes
¼ cup (60 mL) extra virgin olive oil
2 tbsp raw tahini
¼ tsp freshly ground black pepper
1 tsp Himalayan salt
⅛ tsp cayenne pepper
½ tsp freshly ground coriander seeds
1 cup (250 mL) quartered cherry tomatoes

In a food processor, blend all ingredients except tomatoes. Transfer to a serving bowl and mix in tomatoes by hand.

MAKES ABOUT 2 CUPS (500 mL)

A versatile pâté, this can be enjoyed in "sushi" or collard rolls, spread on crackers, or simply eaten as a dip. The toasted sesame oil (which is optional) gives it its Asian flavor.

3 tbsp grated ginger
½ cup (60 mL) chopped red onions
1 cup (250 mL) seeded and chopped red bell peppers
3 cups (750 mL) sunflower seeds, soaked for 6–8 hours
   (reserve soak water)
2 tbsp lemon juice
3 tbsp raw tahini
3 tbsp gluten-free tamari
1 tbsp toasted sesame oil (optional)
cayenne pepper, to taste
¼ cup (60 mL) chopped cilantro

In a food processor, process ginger, onions, and red peppers. Add sunflower seeds and process again. Add remainder of ingredients except cilantro. If mixture is too thick, add 1 tbsp at a time of soaking water to thin. Add cilantro and pulse until combined. Will keep for 1 week in refrigerator.

ITALIAN BASIL TAPENADE

MAKES ABOUT 5 CUPS (1.25 L)

Bold in color and flavor, this lively tapenade makes a
beautiful centerpiece when served on zucchini rounds,
endive, or romaine lettuce leaves.

2 garlic cloves

2 cups (500 mL) sunflower seeds, soaked for
   6–8 hours

½ cup (125 mL) pine nuts, soaked for 30 minutes

2 cups (500 mL) sun-dried tomatoes, soaked for
   30 minutes (reserve soak water)

2 red bell peppers, seeded and chopped

2 tbsp lemon juice

2 tbsp extra virgin olive oil

2 tbsp gluten-free tamari

1 tbsp Italian seasoning

1 tbsp garlic powder

1 tbsp onion powder

freshly ground black pepper, to taste

1 cup (250 mL) loosely packed basil

In a food processor, process garlic, sunflower seeds,
and pine nuts. Add remainder of ingredients except
basil. Blend until smooth, and add soaking water if
mixture is too thick. Add basil and process again.
Season to taste.

*Tomatoes are an integral part of Italian cuisine,
and the sun-dried variety provide a bold flavor,
especially when combined with bell peppers
and fresh basil. Sundried tomatoes add color,
texture, and depth to dishes. The drying process
concentrates the flavor, so a little goes a long
way.*

FIVE-MINUTE GUACAMOLE

MAKES ABOUT 2 CUPS (500 mL)

Serve this Mexican classic with sliced vegetables and dehydrated corn chips as an appetizer or with the Soft Taco Verde (p. 162) or Chili Sin Carne (p. 164).

3 ripe avocados
3 tbsp minced red onions
juice of 1 large lime
½ tsp Himalayan salt, or to taste
¼ cup (60 mL) minced cilantro
1 medium tomato, finely chopped
dash cayenne pepper, to taste

In a bowl, mash avocados with a fork until almost smooth. Stir in remainder of ingredients, and mix to combine well. Season to taste.

▶ *Avocados are often sold while still hard and unripe. Allow them to ripen on your kitchen counter. If you wish to speed up the process, place avocados in a paper bag and leave on the counter. To speed ripening even further, add an apple or banana to the bag. When ripe, store in the refrigerator until needed.*

PICO DE GALLO

MAKES ABOUT 2 CUPS (500 mL)

My hot-blooded Mexican sister-in-law Maru has our family hooked on this extremely potent and cleansing salsa. Get ready for some serious heat—it's *muy picosa!* Serve with dehydrated crackers or corn chips.

4 medium tomatoes, finely chopped
½ cup (125 mL) finely chopped cilantro
2 jalapeño peppers, seeded and minced, or to taste
2 large garlic cloves, pressed or grated
½ cup (125 mL) minced red onions
juice of ½ lime
juice of ½ lemon
1 tbsp extra virgin olive oil (optional)
¼ tsp Himalayan salt, or to taste

In a bowl, combine tomatoes, cilantro, peppers, garlic, and onions. Add lime and lemon juice, olive oil, and season to taste. Let salsa marinate for an hour before serving.

▶ *Onions are rich in quercetin, a plant chemical that helps relieve chest colds and clear up airways. When eaten raw, onions are beneficial to the heart and circulatory system and can reduce high blood pressure.*

MACRO MISO SPREAD

MAKES ABOUT ⅓ CUP (80 mL)

I used to eat this spread regularly when I followed a macrobiotic diet, and I still enjoy it! It's a tasty spread for raw or gluten-free breads and crackers and also delicious daubed on rounds of cucumber.

¼ cup (60 mL) raw tahini

2 tbsp light miso

2 tbsp purified water

2–3 thinly sliced green onions

¼ cup grated carrot (optional)

1 tsp grated fresh ginger

In a bowl, use a spoon to combine tahini, miso, and water. Stir in green onions, carrots, and ginger.

 There are many varieties of miso paste; yellow miso is lighter and sweeter than the savory dark paste. Always choose organic, non-GM miso. I recommend unpasteurized miso, which retains the living enzymes. Gluten-free miso is made from rice or chickpeas.

SOUR KREAM

MAKES ABOUT ¾ CUP (185 mL)

A bowl of my mother's homemade Russian borscht was not complete without a dollop of sour cream. I loved sour cream so much in my youth that I sometimes ate it straight from the container! Here is a creamy, dairy-free version. Serve with Chili Sin Carne (p. 164), Babuschka's Borscht (p. 98), or other soups, or—go ahead—eat with a spoon!

1 cup (250 mL) cashews, soaked for 30 minutes or more

½ cup (125 mL) purified water

1½ tbsp lemon juice

1 tbsp apple cider vinegar

2 tbsp extra virgin olive oil

½ tsp Himalayan salt

In a blender or food processor, blend all ingredients until smooth and creamy. Allow to set in refrigerator.

SOUR KREAM & ONION DIP

MAKES ABOUT 1½ CUPS (375 ML)

An old favorite traditionally made with sour cream and packaged instant onion soup, this contemporary non-dairy dip is guaranteed to impress your friends. Serve with sliced vegetables and dehydrated crackers.

> *I tend to use both garlic and onion powder to round out the flavors in some of these recipes. The powders and granulated (dried) versions are not as intense as fresh garlic or onions, which can sometimes be overbearing.*

2 cups (500 mL) cashews, soaked for 30 minutes or more

1 cup (250 mL) purified water

1 tsp Himalayan salt

2 tsp onion powder

¼ cup (60 mL) extra virgin olive oil

2 tbsp lemon juice

1 tbsp apple cider vinegar

¼ cup (60 mL) granulated onions

1 tbsp extra virgin olive oil, to drizzle

In a blender or food processor, combine all ingredients except granulated onions and garnish. Transfer to a serving bowl and stir in granulated onions. Drizzle with a touch of oil to garnish. **Note:** Dip will thicken after being refrigerated.

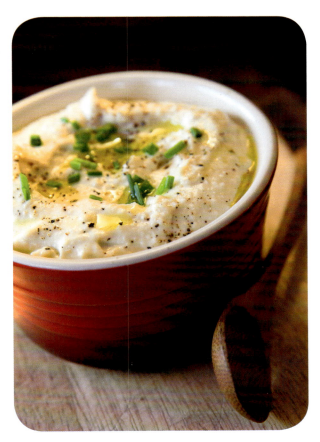

SPINACH & MUSHROOM DIP

This creamy, nutritious party dip makes a delightful appetizer. Serve with a platter of sliced vegetables (baby carrots, diced red and yellow bell peppers, and cauliflower) and dehydrated crackers. It's also delicious as a sauce on zucchini noodles.

MAKES ABOUT 3 CUPS (750 mL)

1 garlic clove

½ cup (125 mL) hemp seeds

6 cups (1.5 L) packed fresh spinach

½ cup (125 mL) raw tahini

¼ cup (60 mL) lemon juice

2 cups (500 mL) sliced mushrooms

½ cup (125 mL) seeded and chopped red bell peppers

½ tsp Himalayan salt

¼ tsp freshly ground black pepper

⅛ tsp ground nutmeg

cayenne pepper, to taste

In a food processor, blend garlic, hemp seeds, and spinach. Add remainder of ingredients one at a time, blending until it reaches a creamy consistency.

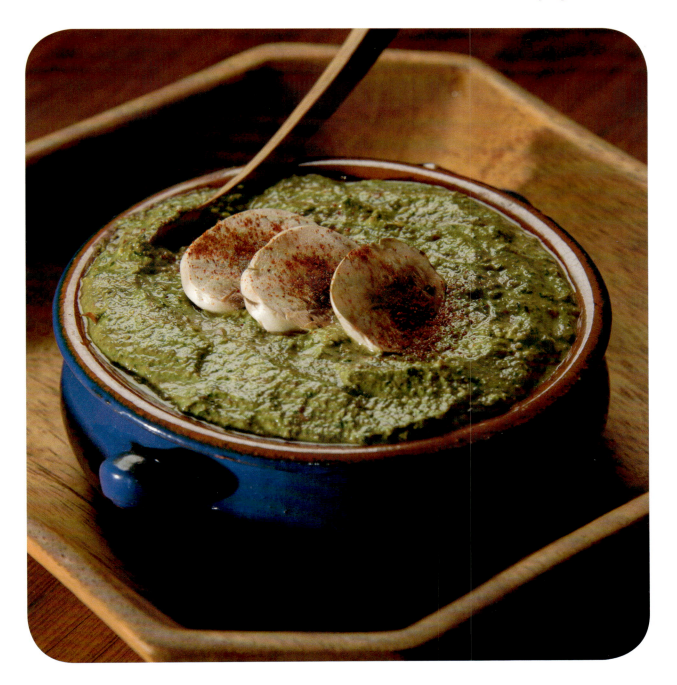

About Cheeze

When I was growing up, I loved eating cheese and often took comfort in it—especially the old, pungent varieties that my Moldavian father brought home. On special occasions, such as Christmas and New Year's Eve, my siblings and I looked forward to eating cheese fondue. With long-stemmed forks, we would dip cubed pieces of French bread into a mixture of melted cheese, wine, and seasonings, kept warm over an open flame. One or two European cheeses were often included in our Sunday lunches. Years later, I continued this tradition while modeling in Germany. In my *pension*, I would put my Swiss Army knife to work, slicing special cheeses, dark rye *brot* (bread), tomatoes, cucumbers, and radishes—a nostalgic picnic accompanied by glass or two of inexpensive wine.

But cheese and other dairy products can be harmful to our health. Cheese has artery-clogging saturated fats and, whether organic or conventional, like all dairy products, it is acidic. Cheese is also high in sodium and contains casein—a protein linked with cancer. Non-organic cheeses can contain residues of toxic pesticides, growth hormones, and antibiotics. (To read more about the relationship between the consumption of animal products and disease, see the book *The China Study* by T. Colin Campbell.)

Because it's so comforting to many people, cheese can be one of the most challenging foods to give up, and many vegans replace it with faux varieties.

Although a step in the right direction, these store-bought imitations are heavily processed and soy-based. Raw vegan cheeze is an entirely different food experience, however; raw nut and seed cheezes are a delicious, healthy substitute for both dairy and soy cheeses. In fact, they taste remarkably similar to dairy cheeses but are made from wholesome, nutritious plant ingredients, prepared by blending nuts and/or seeds to a creamy consistency. Raw vegan cheeze can be prepared quickly or allowed to ferment to create a more flavorful, aged quality.

Cheezes can be made in either a blender or food processor. When blending, you will need to add more water to get the blades moving. Be sure to experiment with various nut, herb, and seasoning combinations to create your own comforting favorites. A block of your homemade nut or seed cheeze served on a bamboo cutting board with grapes, apples, and dehydrated crackers (and perhaps a glass of biodynamic wine) will impress vegans, raw foodists, and cheese connoisseurs alike.

Note: Raw nut and seed cheezes will keep for about 10 days in the refrigerator. They can also be frozen. If you're adding fresh ingredients such as tomatoes, herbs, or onions, the cheeze will keep as long as those ingredients are fresh, generally about 6 days.

SIMPLE CASHEW PINE NUT CHEEZE

MAKES ABOUT 1½ CUPS (375 mL)

If you are prone to cheese cravings, look no further! The recipe can also be made without pine nuts, but they do add an extra richness.

1½ cups (375 mL) cashews, soaked for 30 minutes or more
½ cup (125 mL) pine nuts, soaked for 30 minutes
½ cup (125 mL) purified water
¼ cup (60 mL) lemon juice
¾ tsp Himalayan salt

In a blender or food processor, blend all ingredients on high until completely smooth. Texture should resemble a spreadable cream cheese.

> *Pine nuts are rich and lend an extra creaminess to cheese. You can replace ½ or more cashews with additional pine nuts, or experiment with various nut combinations.*

LEMON DILL CHEEZE

MAKES ABOUT 2½ CUPS (625 mL)

You can really get creative with this cheeze by adding your favorite herbs and spices; try basil, caraway seeds, chipotle, paprika, rosemary, fennel, or oregano. You may also add sun-dried tomatoes, olives, nutritional yeast, and garlic for different flavor combinations. Enjoy with dehydrated crackers, on romaine leaves, or between slices of tomatoes or cucumbers.

3 cups (750 mL) cashews, soaked for 30 minutes or more
½ cup + 2 tbsp lemon juice
¼ cup (60 mL) purified water
1 tbsp extra virgin olive oil
1½ tsp Himalayan salt, or to taste
½ cup (125 mL) fresh chopped dill
1 tbsp dried dill

In a blender or food processor, process cashews with lemon juice until creamy. Gradually add water and blend again. Add remainder of ingredients, in order. Season to taste. (If you don't have fresh dill, use more dried.)

BASIC FERMENTED CHEEZE

MAKES ABOUT 2 CUPS (500 mL)

An all-purpose, rich, and creamy fermented cheeze. I suggest doubling this recipe—it's that good! Enjoy as a spread for crackers, a filling in collard wraps or sushi, or as a dip with veggies.

 Fermenting nuts and seeds is the optimal way to eat them, as they are predigested. Fermented cheezes also have an abundance of valuable enzymes, B vitamins, amino acids, and acidophilus, which helps to balance the natural flora in the intestines. Fermented nut and seed cheezes offer more nutrition for less digestive energy than dairy cheese.

*Adding a few capsules of vegan probiotics is optional, but they do make the cheeze easier to digest. Beneficial bacterial cultures used to speed up the fermentation process in nut cheezes, probiotics are also sold as dietary supplements that contain bacteria naturally occurring in the human intestine (specifically, bifidobacteria and lactic acid bacteria). You can find probiotics in the refrigerated section of most natural food stores. Look for plant-based probiotics. To start the fermentation process, you can also use 1 tbsp miso or Rejuvelac. (My book **The SimplyRaw Living Foods Detox Manual** includes the Rejuvelac recipe.)*

2 cups (500 mL) cashews, soaked for 30 minutes or more
¼ cup (60 mL) lemon juice
½–¾ cup (125–185 mL) purified water, or as needed
¾ tsp Himalayan salt
½ tsp probiotic powder (approximately 3 plant-based probiotic capsules)

In a blender or food processor, blend all ingredients. Gradually add more water if needed to make a smooth mixture. Stop blending and scrape down sides of blender with a spatula, then blend again. Season to taste.

Pour mixture into a sprout bag or cheesecloth-lined colander over a bowl. Wrap cloth to cover and place a weight of about 5 lbs (2.25 kg) on top (I use a large Mason jar filled with water). Place in a warm location and allow to ferment for 24 hours. The longer it ferments, the stronger and tangier the cheeze will taste. (If you want to speed up the process, place in your dehydrator or Infra-red sauna.)

Remove cheeze from cloth and transfer to a bowl. Stir in fresh herbs and spices, if using. Place cheeze into a small ring mould and refrigerate; it will firm up as it chills. Plain fermented cheeze will keep for up to 10 days in the refrigerator, but once fresh herbs are added, the shelf life is shortened.

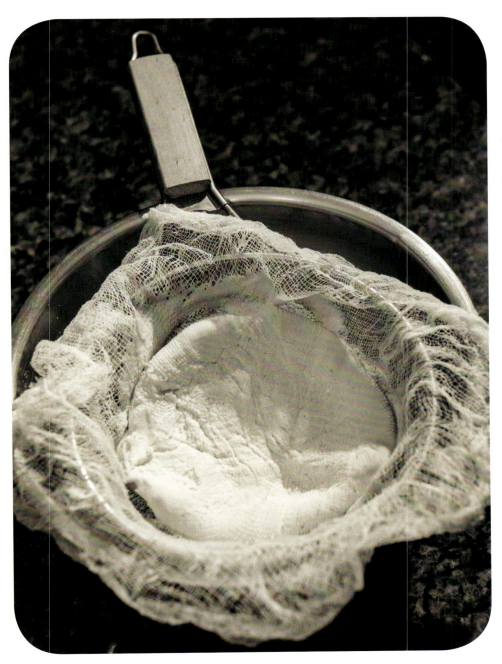

Variation: To develop a rind on the cheeze, place it in a mold and dehydrate (105 °F [41 °C]) for an additional 12–24 hours.

AGED PEPPERCORN CHEEZE

This soft cheese will impress even dairy lovers. If you're in a rush, skip the fermentation process. Serve with dehydrated crackers, grapes, and olives. Yes, miracles do exist!

MAKES ABOUT 2 CUPS (500 ML)

2 cups (500 mL) cashews, soaked for 30 minutes or more

¼ cup (60 mL) lemon juice

½ –¾ cup (125–185 mL) purified water, or as needed

½ tsp probiotic powder (approximately 3 plant-based probiotic capsules)

¾ tsp Himalayan salt

2–3 tsp coarsely ground peppercorns

1–2 tbsp whole peppercorn, for garnish (optional)

In a blender, blend cashews with lemon juice, water, and probiotics until smooth. Add salt and blend again. Add more water if needed to attain a smooth consistency.

Note: If you don't have a blender, in a food processor process cashews, lemon juice, and probiotics with about ½ cup [125 mL] water to make a creamy mixture. Stop processing occasionally and scrape down sides with a spatula. Texture should be thick and smooth.

Pour mixture into a nut mylk bag or cheese-cloth-lined colander over a bowl. Wrap cloth to cover and place a weight of about 5 lbs (2.25 kg) on top. (I use a large Mason jar filled with water.) Place in a warm location and allow to ferment for 24 hours. The longer it ferments, the stronger and tangier the cheeze will taste. (If you want to speed up the process, place in dehydrator or infra-red sauna.)

Once fermented, remove cheeze from cloth and transfer to a bowl, adding coarsely ground peppercorn, mixing until well incorporated. Place cheeze into a small ring mould and garnish with whole peppercorns and refrigerate; it will firm up as it chills. Stored in an airtight container in the refrigerator, cheeze will last up to 10 days.

Variation: To develop a rind on the cheeze, place it in a mold lined with plastic wrap and dehydrate (105°F [41°C]) for an additional 12–24 hours.

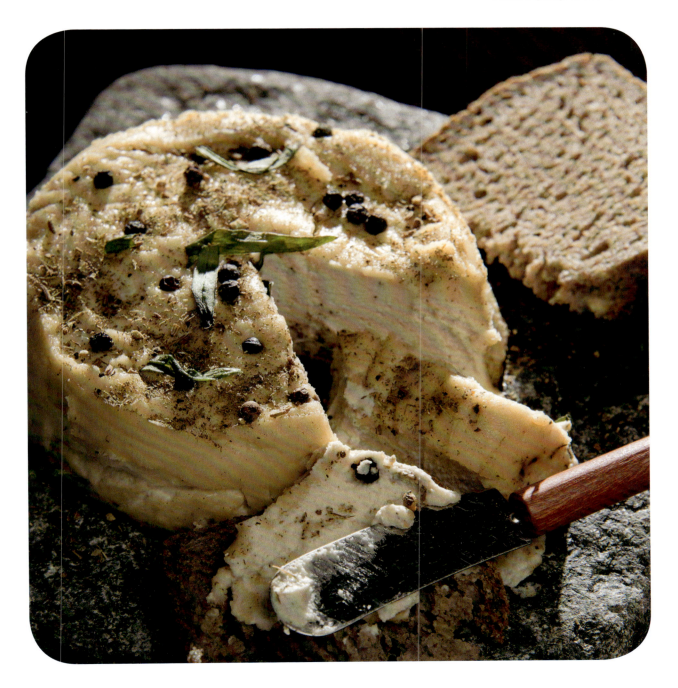

PINE NUT PARMA

MAKES ABOUT ½ CUP (125 mL)

The perfect topping for vegetable pastas, raw chili, or to sprinkle over salads.

¼ cup (60 mL) dry pine nuts

¼ cup (60 mL) dry cashews

⅛ tsp Himalayan salt

½ tsp onion powder

2 tbsp nutritional yeast (optional)

In a food processor, chop nuts to a fine meal (or finely chop by hand). Add salt, onion powder, and yeast and pulse until crumbly. Parma will keep in refrigerator for 1 month.

BASIC ALMOND BUTTER

MAKES ABOUT 2½ CUPS (625 mL)

A simple, delicious recipe that requires only almonds, a food processor, and a whole lot of patience. Make this in advance and store in your refrigerator. Almond butter is delicious on apples, crackers, celery sticks, toast or, once in a while, by the spoonful straight from the jar!

4 cups dry raw almonds

In a food processor, process almonds for about 10 minutes, until smooth. Stop processing occasionally and scrape down sides with a spatula. (Making your own nut butters can put a lot of wear on the processor, so pause several times to avoid overheating the motor.)

Processed almonds will at first appear floury; once oils are released, they will become a creamy, smooth butter. Remember, patience is key. Almond butter will keep for up to 6 months in the refrigerator—as long as you don't add water.

Variations: You can try different nuts (hazelnuts, pecans, cashews, macadamia nuts, walnuts, Brazil nuts, etc.) as well as flavor nut butters with maple syrup, cinnamon, or vanilla.

▶ ***Tip****: If using soaked and dehydrated almonds, ensure that they are thoroughly dried. Don't add water to nut and seed butters; it will reduce shelf life.*

▶ *Almonds grown in the US are now pasteurized in response to isolated incidents of salmonella contamination traced to raw almonds. Although labeled "raw," US almonds (including most raw almond butters) are not truly raw, as they go through a sterilization process using high temperatures to prevent the growth of bacteria. Almonds produced in Spain or Italy do not undergo this process. They are more expensive, but free of chemicals and alive with their natural enzymes. Truly raw almond butters can be found at specialty stores but are very pricey. All the more reason to make your own!*

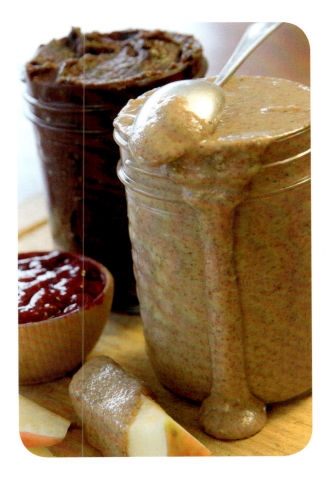

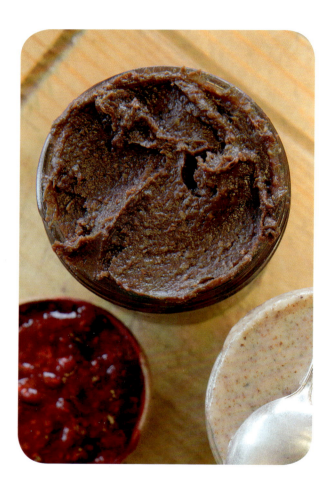

RUSTIC RAWTELLA

MAKES 1¼ CUPS (310 mL)

Super rich and creamy, this coconut-infused Rawtella rivals the decadence of any store-bought chocolate spread!

2 cups (500 mL) dry raw hazelnuts
1–2 tbsp melted coconut oil
2 tsp vanilla extract
¼–½ (60–125 mL) cup maple syrup
¼ cup (60 mL) cacao powder
Himalayan salt, to taste (optional)

In a food processor, process hazelnuts. Stop processing several times and scrape down sides frequently (especially in the beginning), until oils are released, about 10 minutes. Add remainder of ingredients and continue blending until smooth.

HOMEMADE TAHINI

MAKES 2½ CUPS (625 mL)

Tahini is a paste made from ground and hulled sesame seeds. They are an excellent source of calcium, magnesium, iron, zinc, copper, and phosphorous. In ancient Babylon, women were believed to use a mixture of honey and sesame seeds (halva) to prolong youth and beauty, and Roman soldiers ate the mixture for strength and energy.

4 cups (1 L) hulled sesame seeds
2–3 drops sesame oil (optional)

In a food processor, grind seeds. Stop processing occasionally and scrape down sides with a spatula. (Making your own nut butters can put a lot of wear on the processor, so pause several times to avoid overheating the motor.) Continue to process until desired consistency is reached. If after about 12 minutes, sesame seeds have not turned to butter, add sesame oil.

▶ *"Open sesame"—the famous phrase from the Arabian Nights—reflects a distinguishing feature of the sesame seed pod, which bursts open when it reaches maturity.*

HOMEMADE COCONUT BUTTER

MAKES ABOUT 2½ CUPS (625 mL)

A naturally sweet and creamy spread made from blended whole coconut flesh and the oil of coconuts, coconut butter adds a delicious dimension to smoothies, soups, and desserts. Quick, easy, and out of this world!

4 cups shredded organic coconut
1–2 tbsp coconut oil (optional)

In a blender or food processor, blend coconut, stopping occasionally to scrape down sides. At first, coconut flakes will clump; after 5–10 minutes, mixture will start to look smoother; and after 10–20 minutes, it will begin to form a buttery paste. **Tip:** If you wish to speed things along, add 1–2 tbsp coconut oil.

Transfer coconut butter, which will be liquid after blending, to a glass jar. Once cooled, it will solidify. Store in refrigerator. To soften, place in a bowl of hot water until it melts.

▶ *My great aunt "Tanta" Rosa owned a beautiful old inn in the Austrian mountains. When we visited her, she served us home-churned butter spread on dark rye bread for breakfast. It was so thick that my brother and I were convinced it was cheese. (I used a spoon to scoop it off discreetly and fed it to the cat when Rosa wasn't looking!) Coconut oil is a healthy and delicious alternative to dairy butter.*

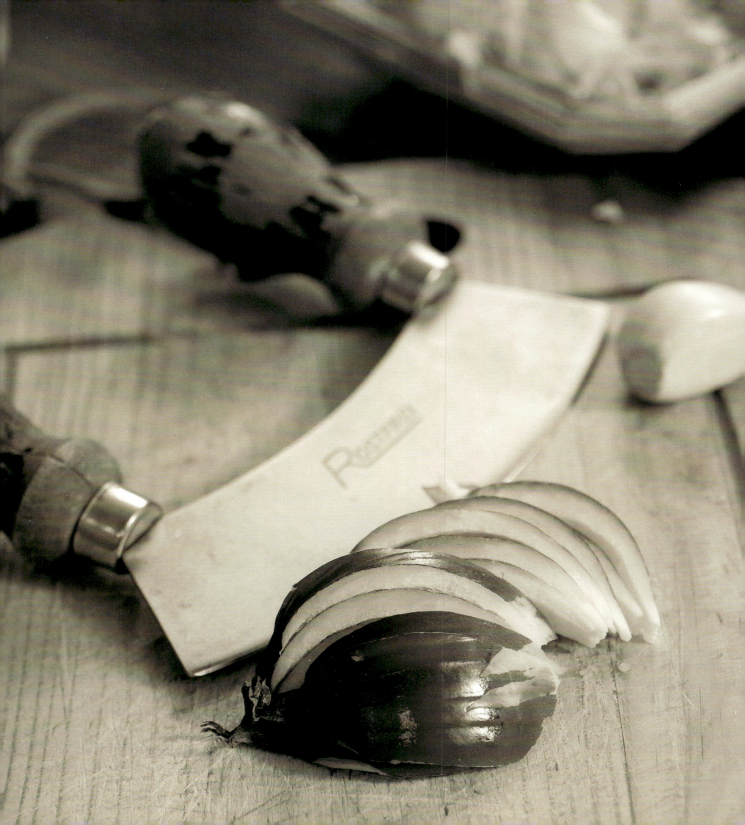

MAINS

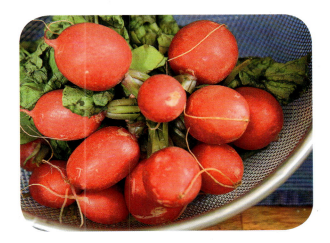

Live It Up Sushi with Ginger Tamari Dipping Sauce   148

Vietnamese Salad Rolls with Dragon Dipping Sauce   150

Happy Hemp Pesto with Parsnip Noodles   152

Kreamy Alfredo with Sweet Potato Noodles 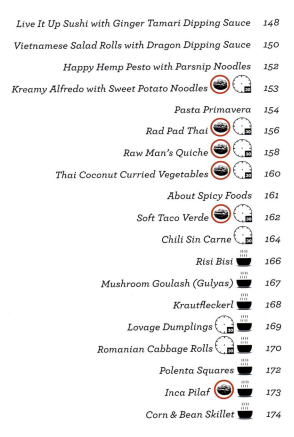   153

Pasta Primavera   154

Rad Pad Thai   156

Raw Man's Quiche   158

Thai Coconut Curried Vegetables   160

About Spicy Foods   161

Soft Taco Verde   162

Chili Sin Carne   164

Risi Bisi   166

Mushroom Goulash (Gulyas)   167

Krautfleckerl   168

Lovage Dumplings   169

Romanian Cabbage Rolls   170

Polenta Squares   172

Inca Pilaf   173

Corn & Bean Skillet   174

What I appreciate most in food (besides good flavor) is simplicity. I like nothing better than a simple salad of ripe tomatoes and cucumbers from the farmer's market or crispy romaine lettuce hearts harvested straight from the earth. Simplicity is also about quality: sourcing high-quality ingredients is by far the most important element of creating a good meal.

Although I discovered the benefits of the raw lifestyle many years ago, I find that my diet has continued to evolve, just as I have. Since turning fifty, I feel best when I eat simpler but nutrient-dense meals; dinners tend to be a blended soup with a side of romaine lettuce and a fermented raw cheeze or an avocado, sauerkraut, and sprouts.

Of course, there are times when we all need

something more filling—raw or cooked—especially in colder climates where we crave warmer foods. Most people find it challenging to eat light all year long. And dinnertime is when most of us want something more substantial, both physically and emotionally. That's why I've included a selection of healthy cooked entrées featuring nourishing, fresh whole plant foods.

The following recipes will inspire you to incorporate more plant foods into your meals. The recipes are simple and realistic, ready for everyday eating. Choose the highest quality ingredients when preparing them. Raw foods don't have to be overly complicated and time-consuming. I am an advocate for dishes that are simple, pure, and nutritious—and I'll show you how to take short cuts in the kitchen wherever possible.

All the recipes have been created to taste so good that it doesn't matter what kind of diet you follow—raw vegan, partially raw, or occasionally raw—you're going to love them!

LIVE IT UP SUSHI WITH GINGER TAMARI DIPPING SAUCE

MAKES 4 NORI ROLLS; EACH ROLL MAKES 6–8 PIECES (2–4 SERVINGS)

This makes a complete meal when accompanied by a bowl of warmed Miso Soup (p. 103). Nori rolls are traditionally eaten with chopsticks, but they also make a fun finger food.

> *I hadn't tasted sushi until I went to Japan on my first modeling contract. Each day, a different client took me to an **ichiban** (number 1) sushi restaurant in Tokyo, and each client had a different favorite. I quickly developed a taste for the fishy stuff, but my raw vegan version is so good that I never miss the original! Making your own sushi may seem intimidating at first, but it's actually quite easy. Before long, you will be making your own creative variations. **Tip**: Use a bamboo sushi mat, which makes it easier to roll.*

4 sheets raw nori

½ recipe Asian Pâté (p. 129)

1½ cups (375 mL) alfalfa sprouts

½ cup (250 mL) shredded carrots

½ red bell pepper, seeded and thinly sliced

1 medium cucumber, seeded and cut lengthwise into 4-in (10-cm) long, thin slices

1 tbsp black sesame seeds, for garnish

On a bamboo sushi mat or cutting board, place 1 nori sheet, shiny side down. Spread ¼ cup (60 mL) pâté evenly across bottom half of nori. Leave about ½ in (1 cm) from bottom and sides of sheet clear. Layer with ½ cup (125 mL) alfalfa sprouts, 2–3 tbsp each shredded carrots and sliced bell peppers, and a few cucumber slices. If you are working on a sushi mat, grasp nori sheet and bottom of mat to help fold nori sheet over filling. Roll up as tightly as possible. To roll without a sushi mat, grasp bottom edge of nori and roll firmly but gently around filling. Moisten edge with water to seal.

With a very sharp knife, cut roll into angled slices. **Tip**: Wipe knife with a cloth between each cut. Arrange slices on a platter and sprinkle with black sesame seeds. Serve with Ginger Tamari Dipping Sauce.

Ginger Tamari Dipping Sauce:

1 tsp ground ginger
¼ cup (60 mL) gluten-free tamari
1 tsp brown rice vinegar
1 tsp maple syrup or 2–3 drops stevia
1 tsp dried wasabi (optional)
2 tbsp minced green onions, for garnish

In a bowl, whisk together all ingredients except green onions. Top with green onions before serving.

▶ *An edible seaweed, nori is often dried into sheets and used to make sushi. It also makes a delicious potato chip substitute, because it has a salty flavor and crisp texture. Nori is a staple in my diet, and because it is also light, I always travel with some.*

▶ *Some raw foodists use coconut aminos, a new alternative to tamari sauce. Although gluten-free, soy-free, and raw, I don't like its chemical taste and prefer to use small amounts of gluten-free tamari.*

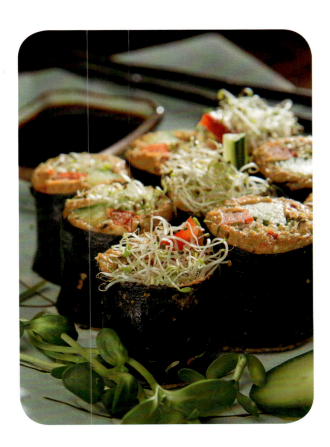

VIETNAMESE SALAD ROLLS WITH DRAGON DIPPING SAUCE

A popular dish at SimplyRaw Express restaurant, these fresh salad rolls are packed with Southeast Asian flavor. The sauce is also good tossed with zucchini or kelp noodles, or as a salad dressing. Make this nut-free by omitting the sauce

MAKES 6 ROLLS (ABOUT 3 SERVINGS)

SAUCE MAKES 1½ CUPS (375 mL)

6 rice wrappers

1½–2 cups (375–500 mL) baby spinach

2 cups (250 mL) julienned red cabbage

1 large mango, peeled, seeded, and sliced

½ red bell peppers, seeded and sliced

½ cup (125 mL) roughly chopped cilantro

¼ cup (60 mL) roughly chopped mint

In a bowl large enough to submerge wrappers, add warm water. Lay a tea towel beside the bowl. Submerge wrappers one at a time until soft, then place on tea towel. Place ½ cup (125 mL) baby spinach at center of wrapper. Top with ¼ cup (60 mL) cabbage. Lay a strip of mango, then a slice of red pepper over cabbage. Top with 1–2 tbsp cilantro and 1 tbsp mint.

Fold sides of wrapper into center. Gently but firmly roll from bottom to top. Place seam-side down on plate.

Rolls may stick to each other, so leave space between them. Serve with a bowl of Dragon Dipping Sauce.

Dragon Dipping Sauce:

3 tbsp lime juice

2 tsp chopped fresh ginger

1 garlic clove

1 red Thai chili pepper (with seeds)

2 tbsp gluten-free tamari

2 tbsp maple syrup or 2–3 pitted Medjool dates

¼ cup (60 mL) + 1 tbsp almond butter

½ cup (125 mL) purified water

½ tbsp melted coconut oil

In a blender or food processor, blend all ingredients except coconut oil until smooth. Add coconut oil and briefly blend again. Don't over-blend. Sauce will thicken once refrigerated. Add 2–4 tbsp water to thin if necessary before serving.

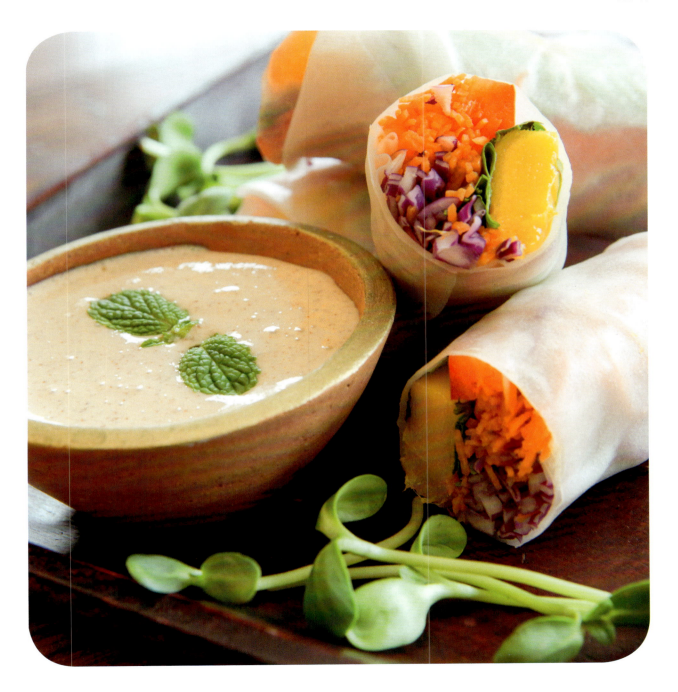

HAPPY HEMP PESTO WITH PARSNIP NOODLES

MAKES 6 SERVINGS

Hemp seeds increase the nutritional value of this delicious, protein- and omega-rich pesto. It is especially appetizing on parsnip noodles (or pasta of your choice) and spread on thickly sliced tomatoes sprinkled with Pine Nut Parma (p. 140).

Noodles:

6–8 large peeled parsnips, spiralized into noodles
1 red bell pepper, seeded and minced
freshly ground black pepper, to taste
3 tbsp finely chopped basil leaves, for garnish
3 tbsp Pine Nut Parma (p. 140), for garnish (optional)

In a large bowl, combine spiralized parsnips with bell peppers and set aside.

Pesto:

4–5 garlic cloves
½ cup (125 mL) sundried tomatoes, soaked for 30 minutes
5–6 cups packed chopped spinach
1 cup (250 mL) packed fresh basil
½ cup (125 mL) hemp seeds
2 tbsp lemon juice
½ cup (125 mL) extra virgin olive oil
2 tbsp gluten-free tamari
3 tbsp nutritional yeast (optional)
⅛ tsp freshly ground black pepper
cayenne pepper, to taste
1 tsp Himalayan salt

In a food processor, process garlic and sundried tomatoes. Add spinach and process until smooth. Add remainder of pesto ingredients one at a time, and blend until fairly smooth. Toss pesto with noodles and red peppers. Sprinkle with freshly ground black pepper, basil, and Pine Nut Parma. Happy Hemp Pesto freezes well.

Rich in B vitamins, nutritional yeast lends a cheesy flavor to many recipes. It tastes wonderful when sprinkled on air-popped popcorn drizzled with flax oil and a pinch of Himalayan salt and cayenne pepper. Nutritional yeast is fortified with B12—which makes it a valuable food for vegans.

KREAMY ALFREDO
WITH SWEET POTATO NOODLES

MAKES 4–6 SERVINGS;
SAUCE MAKES ABOUT 2 CUPS [500 mL]

This dish has such a creamy texture and taste, you'll never miss traditional cheesy pasta again!

Noodles:

2 medium sweet potatoes, peeled and spiralized

2 cups (250 mL) bite-sized broccoli florets

½ cup (125 mL) sliced white mushrooms

¼ cup (60 mL) finely chopped parsley, for garnish

Alfredo Sauce:

½ cup (125 mL) purified water

1 garlic clove

½ cup (125 mL) red bell pepper

1 cup (250 mL) cashews, soaked for 30 minutes or more

3 tbsp lemon juice

2 tbsp gluten-free tamari

3 tbsp extra virgin olive oil

2 tbsp nutritional yeast

½ tsp Himalayan salt

¼ tsp ground turmeric

½ tsp dried rosemary

½ tsp paprika

cayenne pepper, to taste

⅛ tsp freshly ground black pepper

Toss spiralized sweet potatoes with broccoli, and mushrooms. For sauce; in a blender, blend water with garlic and bell peppers. Add remainder of ingredients and blend until creamy. Pour sauce over noodles and vegetables, and toss to combine well. Season to taste. Garnish with parsley.

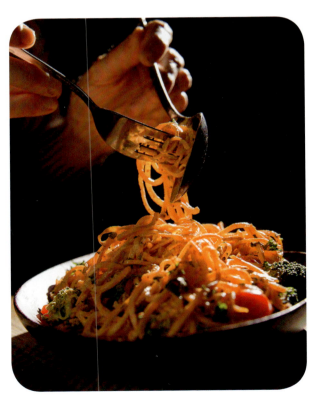

PASTA PRIMAVERA

The most delicious and satisfying meals are often the simplest. This flavorful favorite is bound to sweep you away. Make it your very own low-carb staple. Enjoy with a glass of biodynamic red wine, if you wish. Bellissima!

MAKES 4 SERVINGS

> *Italy is my favorite European country for its passionate people, fascinating history, art, culture, and, of course, its excellent food. In Italy, pasta is a staple. This raw adaptation has been my stand-by meal for years. It never fails to transport me back to Piazza Navona in Rome, where my waiter sang to me over dinner.*

Noodles:

6 medium zucchinis, peeled

freshly ground black pepper, to taste

2 tbsp chopped fresh basil, for garnish

2–3 tbsp Pine Nut Parma (p. 142), for garnish (optional)

Slice zucchini in thirds, then spiralize into thin noodles. Set in colander to drain. (See sidebar, opposite; this step is optional but recommended.)

Primavera Sauce:

4 medium Roma tomatoes, chopped

1 cup (250 mL) chopped red bell peppers

2 garlic cloves

1 cup (250 mL) sun-dried tomatoes, soaked for 30 minutes

2 tbsp pitted Kalamata olives

1 tsp lemon juice

2 tbsp extra virgin olive oil

2 pitted Medjool dates or 1 tbsp maple syrup

2 tsp onion powder

1 tsp garlic powder

1 tsp Italian seasoning

3 tbsp minced fresh basil leaves

1 tbsp minced fresh oregano leaves

1 tbsp gluten-free tamari

⅛ tsp freshly ground black pepper

cayenne pepper, to taste

In a blender, blend tomatoes, red pepper, and garlic. Add remainder of sauce ingredients and blend until well mixed. Spoon over noodles and sprinkle with black pepper, basil, and Pine Nut Parma (optional).

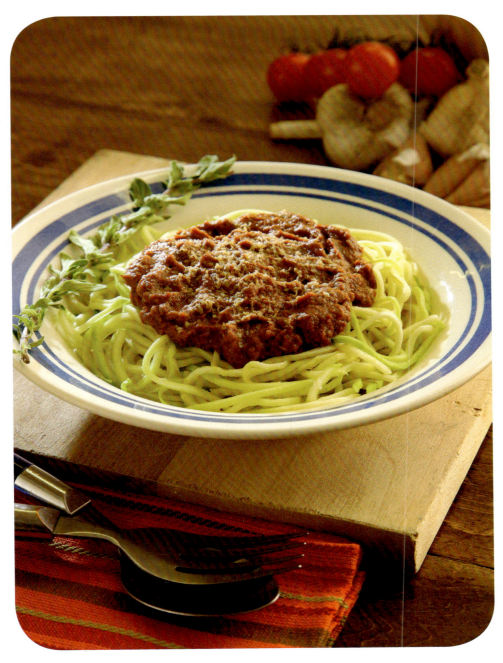

Once zucchini noodles are mixed with sauce, they will release a lot of water, making them soggy. Drain spiralized noodles in a colander, sprinkled with a little salt, before adding sauce. Or pat zucchini between paper towels to pull out some of the excess moisture.

RAD PAD THAI

My magical year of living in a thatched hut in Thailand inspired this delicious dish with authentic Thai flavor. Escape to an exotic land right in your own kitchen.

MAKES 4–6 SERVINGS

SAUCE MAKES 1½ CUPS [375 mL]

Noodles:

6 medium zucchinis

¼ cup (60 mL) finely sliced red cabbage

1 small carrot, julienned

½ cup (125 mL) chopped fresh cilantro

1 green onion, thinly sliced, for garnish

2 tbsp basil, chopped, for garnish

2 quartered Roma tomatoes

½ lime, quartered

Slice zucchini into thirds, then spiralize into thin noodles. Transfer to a large mixing bowl and top with cabbage, carrots, and cilantro. Set aside while you make sauce.

Sauce:

¼ cup (60 mL) lime juice

1 tbsp chopped fresh ginger

1 garlic clove

2 tbsp gluten-free tamari

2 tbsp maple syrup

¼ cup (60 mL) chopped Roma tomatoes

⅓ cup (80 mL) purified water

¼ cup (60 mL) almond butter

1 tbsp sun-dried tomatoes, soaked for 30 minutes

1 tbsp coconut oil

In a blender, blend all sauce ingredients except coconut oil until smooth. Add coconut oil and briefly blend again. Pour sauce over vegetables and toss to combine well. Top with green onions and basil. Serve with quartered Roma tomatoes on the side and lime to squeeze over top.

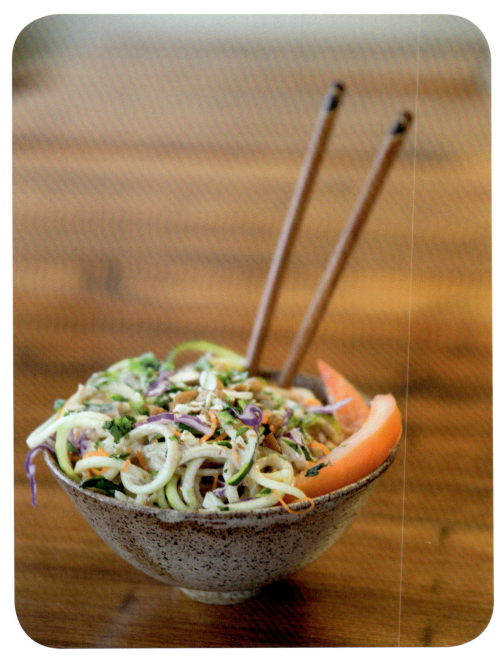

Note: *The sauce will thicken once refrigerated. If you are serving it right away, use less water. It is also delicious on kelp noodles, a low-calorie, gluten-free, raw substitute for pasta. Made from the sea vegetable kelp, sodium alginate (seaweed-derived salt), and water, kelp noodles are a good source of minerals and iodine, which is essential for proper thyroid function. To use, simply rinse under water and drain. Because their flavor is neutral, they pick up the taste of whatever they are mixed with. Their texture is mildly crunchy, but surprisingly like al dente pasta.*

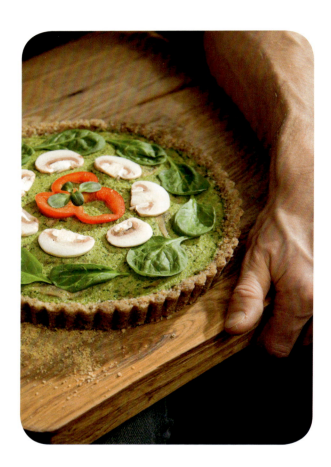

RAW MAN'S QUICHE

MAKES 6–8 SERVINGS

This version of the quintessential brunch food is packed with more than enough clean protein to fuel any man. Who says real men don't eat quiche?

Crust:

3 cups (750 mL) dry walnuts

¼ cup (60 mL) ground golden flax seeds

½ tsp dried *herbes de Provence*

1 tbsp gluten-free tamari

1 tbsp water (optional)

Marinated Mushrooms:

2 cups (500 mL) finely sliced mushrooms

2 tbsp extra virgin olive oil

2 tbsp gluten-free tamari

⅛ tsp freshly ground black pepper

Filling:

2 garlic cloves

1½ cups (375 mL) cashews, soaked 30 minutes or more

½ cup (125 mL) pine nuts, soaked 30 minutes or more

¼ cup (60 mL) lemon juice

2 tbsp extra virgin olive oil

3 tbsp nutritional yeast

2 tbsp gluten-free tamari

1½ tsp onion powder

½ tsp freshly ground coriander seeds

1 tsp dried *herbes de Provence*

¼ tsp cayenne pepper

6 cups (1.5 L) packed chopped spinach

2 tbsp psyllium husk

freshly ground black pepper and Himalayan salt, to
taste

In a food processor, process crust ingredients until
dough sticks together. Press into an 8-in (20-cm)
springform pan or pie plate with a removable bottom.
Place mushrooms, olive oil, tamari, and black pepper
in a medium bowl. Massage mushrooms to soften
them, then set aside.

To make filling, in a food processor, process garlic
until crushed. Add cashews, pine nuts, lemon juice,
olive oil, nutritional yeast, tamari, onion powder,
coriander, *herbes de Provence*, and cayenne pepper
and blend until smooth. Add spinach and mushroom
marinade liquid, and blend again. Add psyllium husks
and pulse briefly. Transfer to a medium bowl and stir
to combine well. Season to taste. Spoon onto crust
and decorate with mushrooms.

*Psyllium is a good source of soluble fiber and is
also used as a thickener in many raw recipes.*

*Massaging vegetables softens them without the
need to cook them. This preserves both nutrients
and enzymes, which are depleted by heat, as well
as time.*

THAI COCONUT CURRIED VEGETABLES

MAKES 6 SERVINGS

This delicate Thai-style curry is mild yet full of flavor. Curry is a blend of warming spices, which makes this dish especially comforting during the cold months. Serve on raw baby spinach or cooked quinoa.

> *Turmeric contains powerful antioxidant properties used in the treatment of various ailments including inflammation, digestive disorders, and liver disease.*

Curry Sauce:

1 cup (250 mL) cashews, soaked for 30 minutes

1 cup (250 mL) purified water

2 tbsp minced red onions

¼ cup (60 mL) chopped tomatoes

1 garlic clove

1 tbsp grated ginger

3 tbsp melted coconut butter or shredded dried coconut

2 tbsp curry powder

⅛ tsp ground turmeric

1 kaffir lime leaf

1½ tsp Himalayan salt

2 tbsp lime juice

2–3 pitted Medjool dates

1 tbsp melted coconut oil

cayenne pepper, to taste

Vegetables:

8 cups (2 L) cauliflower, cut into small pieces

2 cups (500 mL) diced carrots

3 cups (750 mL) fresh or frozen peas

1 cup (250 mL) halved cherry tomatoes

1 cup (250 mL) diced orange, yellow, or red bell peppers

1 cup (250 mL) Thompson raisins

¼ cup chopped cilantro, for garnish

In a blender or food processor, blend all sauce ingredients until smooth. In a medium bowl, combine all vegetables. Top with sauce and toss to combine well. Garnish with cilantro.

About Spicy Foods

It's a myth that spicy food aggravates ulcers and other stomach ailments. Research shows that hot peppers, which contain the anti-inflammatory capsaicin, can protect a healthy stomach lining, and eating hot peppers may prevent gastric damage. There's also evidence that chilies can reduce the risk of cardiovascular disease and boost metabolism.

You don't need to be a heat fiend to appreciate the benefits of hot spices. Cultures around the world have been using them medicinally for thousands of years. Now, research is proving the power of hot chilies as effective painkillers; they are also an excellent source of vitamin A and help to boost immunity. Their active ingredient capsaicin is being studied in cancer treatments and as a regulator for blood sugar levels.

Chipotles are jalapeño peppers that have been dried and smoked. Since the jalapeño's thick flesh does not dry quickly in the sun and is prone to deterioration, a smoke-drying process, also used to preserve meat, was adapted to preserve the chilies. The name "chipotle" comes from the Nahuatl word *chilpoctli*, meaning smoked chili pepper. Chipotles are known for their bold, lively heat and smoky flavor and are available whole or ground. I buy them whole and grind them in my coffee grinder (reserved for spices) or by hand in a mortar and pestle.

In my family, we have a long-standing tradition of eating a lot of very hot, spicy foods. A serious lover of hot chilies, my father frequently challenged us in games of culinary masochism to see who could eat the spiciest foods!

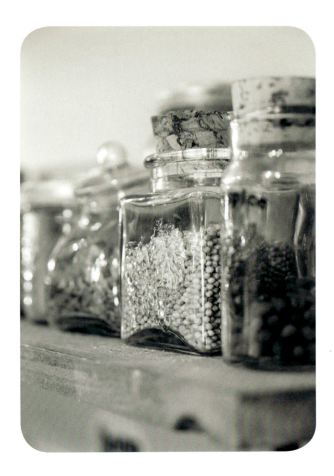

SOFT TACO VERDE

Comforting and flavorful, this Mexican delight is sure to satisfy everyone's appetite.
Serve with Five-Minute Guacamole (p. 131) to complete the Mexican theme.

MAKES 4–5 TACOS

Taco "Shells":

4–5 red or green cabbage leaves

Walnut "Neat":

2 cups (500 mL) dry walnuts

1 tbsp gluten-free tamari

2 tsp onion powder

1 tsp garlic powder

2 tsp ground cumin

½ tsp ground coriander seeds

¼ tsp paprika

½ tsp ground chipotle peppers or chili powder, or to taste

dash freshly ground black pepper

1 tbsp extra virgin olive oil

Himalayan salt, to taste

2 cups (500 mL) chopped romaine lettuce leaves

½ cup (125 mL) quartered cherry tomatoes

½ cup (125 mL) Sour Kream (p. 132)

1 lime, quartered

Optional: Soak walnuts for 8 hours and dehydrate for 12–14 hours, or use raw dry walnuts.

In a food processor, lightly pulse walnuts, tamari, onion powder, garlic powder cumin, coriander, paprika, chipotle, black pepper, and oil until crumbly. Do not over-blend or it will become too oily. Season to taste.

On a plate, lay 1 cabbage leaf. Add 2 heaping tbsp of taco filling. Top with ¼ cup (60 mL) romaine and 2 tbsp cherry tomatoes. Add more walnut mixture, then top with Sour Kream and Guacamole. Serve with a wedge of lime that can be squeezed over the taco.

 If you don't have a dehydrator, use dry raw walnuts for a next-to-best option.

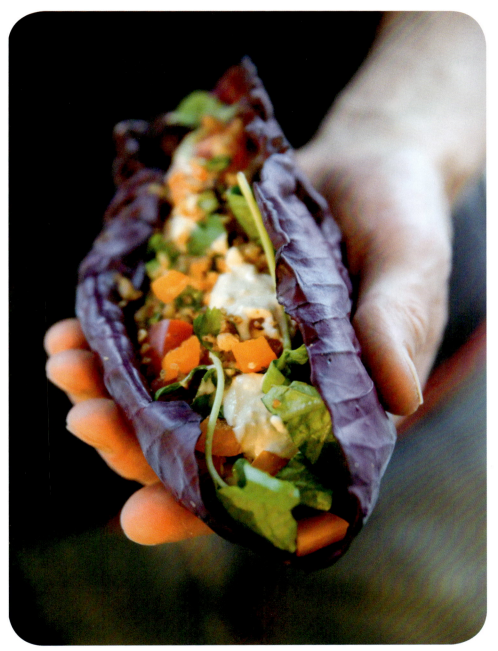

Variations: *For taco shells, you can also use Napa cabbage leaves, romaine lettuce leaves, dehydrated raw corn taco shells, or sprouted organic corn shells.*

CHILI SIN CARNE

Nothing says comfort like a hearty bowl of chili in the middle of winter. This dish is an updated raw vegan version of old-fashioned meat or soy chili. The flavors are a perfect blend of tomatoes, garlic, and spices. Serve it with Sour Kream (p. 132), Guacamole (p. 131), and Polenta Squares (p. 172) or a baked gluten-free bun.

MAKES 6–8 SERVINGS

Chili:

1 medium carrot, grated

1 celery stalk, diced

1 red bell pepper, seeded and diced

1 yellow bell pepper, seeded and diced

1 medium zucchini, diced

¼ medium red onion, minced

2 Portobello mushrooms, finely chopped

1 cup (250 mL) fresh or frozen corn

3 tbsp lemon juice

1 tsp Himalayan salt

3 tbsp extra virgin olive oil

In a large bowl, combine vegetables for chili and massage lightly with lemon juice, salt, and oil.

Chili Sauce:

¼ cup (60 mL) purified water

1½ cups (375 mL) sun-dried tomatoes, soaked for 30 minutes

4 medium Roma tomatoes, chopped

2 small garlic cloves

¼ cup (60 mL), extra virgin olive oil

1 tbsp lemon juice

3 tbsp gluten-free tamari

1 tsp dried basil

1 tsp dried oregano

1 tsp ground cumin

1 tsp onion powder

1 tsp garlic powder

1 pitted Medjool date

3 tbsp chili powder

1 tsp ground chipotle pepper

dash cayenne pepper

¼ cup (60 mL) finely chopped cilantro for garnish

In a blender, blend all sauce ingredients until smooth. Stir into vegetables and allow flavors to meld for 1 hour. If desired, dehydrate at 105°F (41°C) or, in a large pot on low heat, lightly warm on stove. Serve garnished with cilantro.

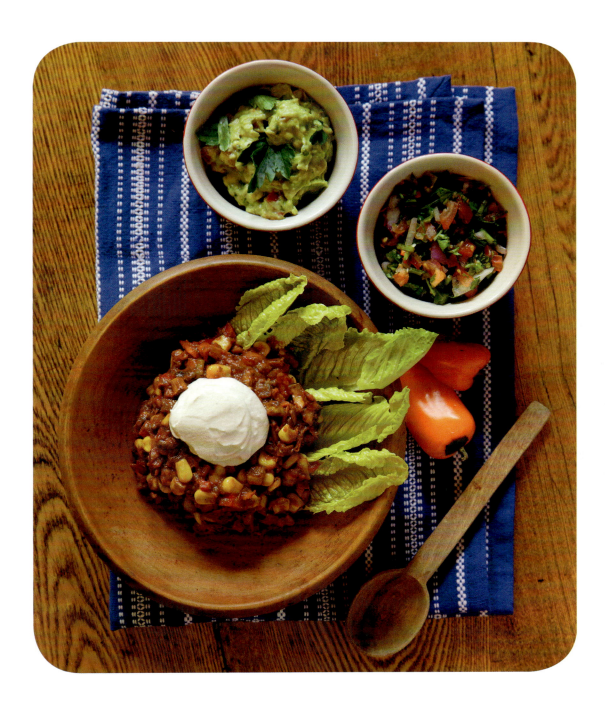

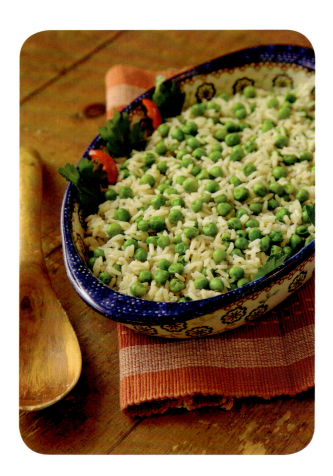

RISI BISI

MAKES 2–4 SERVINGS

My mother has been serving this simple rice and pea dish for decades, and it's still a family favorite, especially with her grandchildren—my teenaged son loves his Omi's Risi Bisi! Serve with a salad for a quick, easy, and hearty dinner.

2 cups (500 mL) purified water

1 tsp Himalayan salt

1 slice onion, studded with 2 whole cloves

1 cup (250 mL) brown basmati rice, well rinsed

1 tbsp extra virgin olive oil

2 cups (500 mL) fresh or frozen green peas, steamed
   for 5 minutes

1 tsp dried basil

½ cup (125 mL) minced parsley, for garnish

In a medium pot on high heat, bring water, salt, and onion with cloves to a boil. Add rice and reduce heat to low. Cover pot and let simmer for about 25 minutes, until water is absorbed. Remove onion and gently mix in peas and basil. Serve topped with plenty of fresh parsley.

 Rich in vitamins A and C, parsley is a great herb to include in your daily diet. It helps to cleanse the liver and spleen, is a diuretic, and refreshes the breath.

MUSHROOM GOULASH (GULYAS)

MAKES 2–3 SERVINGS

In Austria, goulash comes in many varieties—potato, pumpkin, mushroom, and meat. It is usually accompanied by dumplings, noodles, plain polenta, or a fresh *Semmel* (roll or bun). My mother's hearty and satisfying goulash made a regular appearance at our supper table when I was growing up. Although she won't admit it, I am sure that she added a few tablespoons of wine for flavor!

2 cups (500 mL) diced onions

1 medium tomato, chopped

1 small carrot, diced

1 small red bell pepper, diced

1 tsp dried marjoram

1 tsp dried thyme

1 tsp ground caraway seeds

1 tsp Himalayan salt

1 tbsp Hungarian paprika

1 bay leaf

1 piece of lemon peel

3 cups (750 mL) sliced mushrooms

1 large garlic clove, pressed or grated

1 tbsp arrowroot powder mixed with enough cold water to form a smooth paste

2 tbsp white wine (optional)

⅛ tsp cayenne pepper

In a large saucepan, braise onions in ½ cups (125 mL) water until golden and softened. Add tomato, carrots, bell peppers, herbs, caraway seeds, salt, paprika, bay leaf, and lemon zest, and braise for 3 minutes. Stir frequently to prevent burning. Stir in mushrooms and add 1 cup (250 mL) boiling water. Cover pot and cook for about 20 minutes, stirring frequently. Remove lemon peel. Add garlic and arrowroot paste and cook for another 3 minutes. Stir in wine, if using, and cayenne pepper, and season to taste.

"The onion has long been praised for its health benefits. The sulfur-containing compound in onions stimulates the immune system and fights invading germs. When I was growing up, we used to put sliced raw onions in saucers in every room in the house during flu season; the onions were believed to absorb germs in the air. When my 95-year-old grandmother was coming down with a cold, she would put raw sliced onions into the woolen socks she wore to bed; the next morning, she felt fine and went back to her daily chores."
—Ilse

KRAUTFLECKERL

MAKES 3–5 SERVINGS

Caraway seeds are one of the most important spices in Austrian cooking; a kitchen is not a kitchen without them. The seeds were believed to have magical powers and were used in love potions. In Austria, they are also used extensively in cabbage and potato dishes, breads, salt-baked goods, cheeses, sauerkraut, and *Kümmel*, an after-dinner digestive liqueur.

1 small onion, finely chopped

1 tbsp coconut sugar

1 small tomato, diced

1 tbsp ground caraway seeds

1 tsp dried savory

1 small green cabbage, finely chopped (about
   5 cups [1.25 L])

1 tbsp extra virgin olive oil

1 tsp Himalayan salt

2 cups (500 mL) cooked gluten-free small pasta
   (macaroni or bowties)

freshly ground black pepper, to taste

In a large pot on medium-low heat, braise onions and sugar in ½ cup (125 mL) purified water for about 5 minutes, stirring constantly. Add tomatoes, caraway seeds, and savory, and cook for another 2–3 minutes

before adding cabbage, oil, and salt. Stir to combine well. Add 1 cup (250 mL) boiling water and cover pot. Cook over medium heat for about 30 minutes, adding more water if needed to prevent burning, until cabbage is tender and water absorbed. Remove from heat and stir in pasta. Garnish with freshly ground black pepper.

> *"Instead of using commercial pasta in her Krautfleckerl, my mother used small pieces of cooked dough called* **Fleckerl***, meaning 'little rags.'"* —Ilse

> *Caraway is an ancient spice known to traders along the Silk Road. The seeds are beneficial to the stomach, aid digestion, and have a pleasant aromatic essence.*

LOVAGE DUMPLINGS

MAKES 16 SMALL DUMPLINGS

Lovage is a plant that resembles and tastes like wild celery but has a warm, spicy fragrance. Young, finely chopped leaves can be added to salads, but should be used sparingly because of their strong flavor. Serve these dumplings as a side dish with Goulash (p. 167).

1 cup (250 mL) chickpea flour

1 tsp Himalayan salt

3 tbsp ground flaxseeds soaked in ½ cup (125 mL) water for 30 minutes

2 tbsp crumbled dried lovage leaves or 1 cup finely chopped fresh leaves

½ tsp dried thyme

1 tbsp extra virgin olive oil

freshly ground black pepper, to taste

¼ cup (60 mL) finely chopped parsley

In a large bowl, combine all ingredients except parsley. Stir with a wooden spoon to combine well and let rest for 15 minutes.

Meanwhile, in a large pot on high heat, bring about 10 cups (2.5 L) purified water to a boil with a pinch of salt and a drop of oil.

Dip a teaspoon into a glass of cold water, then scoop 1 tsp dough and drop into boiling water. Wet spoon in cold water before each scoop. Reduce heat to medium and cook dumplings for 10–15 minutes, until they rise to surface. Remove with a slotted spoon, transfer to a colander, and rinse under cold water. In a large frying pan on medium, heat 2–3 tbsp water and add parsley. Add dumplings, stir to coat well, and serve hot.

 *This is a savory variation of traditional Austrian **Nockerl** (dumplings), made from butter, milk, egg, and white flour. In folk medicine, tea from the lovage root was used as a cure for rheumatism and stomach disorders. Lovage leaves were put into shoes to revive weary travelers, and a lovage cordial was served in rural inns and considered very beneficial to health.*

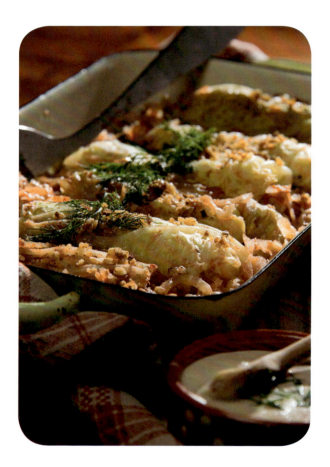

ROMANIAN CABBAGE ROLLS ♨

MAKES 6 SERVINGS

I loved cabbage rolls as a child, and when I was pregnant, often dreamed about them! This dish makes a baker's dozen (13) rolls and tastes even better when reheated the following day. Serve these as is or garnished with a dollop of Sour Kream (p. 132).

1½ cups (375 mL) purified water
½ tsp Himalayan salt
¾ cup (185 mL) uncooked buckwheat

In a pot on high heat, bring water and salt to a boil. Add buckwheat, reduce heat to low, and cook for 20 minutes. Set aside.

1¼ cups (310 mL) purified water
½ tsp Himalayan salt
¾ cup (185 mL) uncooked quinoa

In a separte pot on medium heat bring water and salt to a boil. Add quinoa, reduce heat to low, and cook for 20 minutes. Set aside.

1 tbsp gluten-free tamari
1 tbsp nutritional yeast
1 tsp dried basil

1 tsp dried thyme

½ tsp dried savory

½ tsp dried marjoram

1 tbsp extra virgin olive oil

1 tsp Himalayan salt, or to taste

⅛ tsp cayenne pepper

1 small onion, finely chopped

1 large garlic clove, pressed or grated

1 cup (250 mL) finely chopped sundried tomatoes

1 large Savoy cabbage

2 cups (500 mL) tomato juice

2 cups (500 mL) sauerkraut

½ cup (125 mL) chopped fresh dill, for garnish

In a large bowl, combine cooked buckwheat and quinoa with tamari, nutritional yeast, herbs, oil, salt, and cayenne and set aside.

In a medium frying pan, braise onions, garlic, and sundried tomatoes in ½ cup (125 mL) water for 5 minutes, stirring constantly until water is absorbed. Stir into buckwheat mixture.

Carefully detach about 13 cabbage leaves. In a large covered pot, on medium heat, steam leaves for about 2 minutes, until lightly wilted, then drain.

On a cutting board, place one leaf at a time and fill with 1–2 tbsp of buckwheat mixture, depending on size of leaf. Tuck in sides and roll leaf neatly upward so filling does not spill out. Repeat until all filling has been used.

Divide 1 cup (250 mL) tomato juice between 2 large frying pans. Place cabbage rolls seam-side down in juice. Place sauerkraut between rolls. Pour remainder of juice over rolls and cover pans. On medium-low heat, cook for 15–20 minutes. Baste cabbage rolls with juice a few times. Garnish with dill.

▶ *Because my father was Eastern European, cabbage was always a staple in our household. My mother cooked it in soups, made cabbage rolls with it, grated it in salads, or simmered it with apples. But this traditional hearty peasant food doesn't get the respect it deserves in North America. Not only is it economical, cabbage is highly nutritious, rich in vitamins A, C, and K, and the minerals potassium, calcium, and magnesium. Cabbage-based salads stay fresh longer than those made with lettuce.*

POLENTA SQUARES

MAKES 4–6 SERVINGS

Polenta is popular in Southern Austria, near the Slovenian border. This versatile cornmeal dish can be served soft or firm and shaped into squares or triangles. Serve Polenta Squares with Chili Sin Carne (p. 164) and salad for a complete meal.

 "I often had polenta for breakfast as a child. It was called 'the poor man's food' because the ingredients were so inexpensive. My father liked to eat it with mushroom soup, my mother had it with barley coffee, and I enjoyed it with elderberry jam and cinnamon." —Ilse

1 cup (250 mL) minced kale

6 finely chopped sundried tomatoes, soaked for 30 minutes

1 tbsp extra virgin olive oil

½ tsp Himalayan salt

½ tsp dried basil

½ tsp ground cumin

1 tsp dried sage leaves

1 garlic clove, grated or pressed

⅛ tsp cayenne pepper

1 tsp Himalayan salt

1¼ cups (310 mL) cornmeal

2 tbsp dry sunflower or pumpkin seeds

Preheat oven to 450°F (230°C).

In a large cast iron pan on medium heat, braise kale and sundried tomatoes in ½ cup (125 ml) water, until water is absorbed. Stir in oil, ½ tsp salt, basil, cumin, sage, garlic, and cayenne pepper, and set aside.

In a medium pot on high heat, bring 3 cups (750 mL) water with 1 tsp salt to a boil. Reduce heat to medium and slowly add cornmeal in a steady stream. Reduce heat to low and whisk mixture constantly to prevent lumps from forming. Cover pot and continue to cook on very low heat, stirring frequently, for about 10 minutes.

Stir cooked kale mixture into cornmeal and blend well. Sprinkle with sunflower or pumpkin seeds. Transfer to an 11- x 7-in (2-L) lightly oiled casserole dish and bake on middle rack in oven for 15 minutes. Broil for about 3 minutes, until golden brown. Cut into squares or triangles to serve.

 "An old proverb says, 'How can a man die who has sage in his garden?'

Sage is known for its many healing properties. Made into a tea, the leaves are said to reduce night sweats and hot flashes. As a gargle, sage can soothe a sore throat. When burned, the odor helps to clear impurities from a room. Sage tea is said to stop the flow of milk in nursing mothers. Sage wine and ale are used as nerve and blood tonics. And the leaves of this slightly bitter herb deter moths from damaging linens." —Ilse

INCAN PILAF

MAKES ABOUT 2–4 SERVINGS

Quinoa has been cultivated for thousands of years. It is a complete protein, containing all the amino acids. Tasty and easy to digest, it's also quick to prepare.

1½ cups (125 mL) water

1 tsp Himalayan salt

1 cup (250 mL) uncooked quinoa

1 small onion, finely chopped

½ cup (125 mL) diced red bell peppers

½ cup (125 mL) currants, soaked in ½ cup
   (125 mL) water for 10 minutes (reserve soak water)

½ cup (125 mL) dried cranberries soaked in ½ cup
   (125 mL) water for 10 minutes (reserve soak water)

¼ tsp ground allspice

¼ tsp ground cloves

¼ tsp ground cinnamon

¼ tsp ground cumin

¼ tsp dried thyme

1 tsp ground ginger

½ cup (125 mL) lightly toasted slivered almonds

3 green onions, finely sliced

⅛ tsp cayenne pepper

½ tsp Himalayan salt

1 tbsp extra virgin olive oil

½ cup chopped dry pumpkin seeds, for garnish

In a large saucepan on high heat, bring water and 1 tsp salt to a boil. Add quinoa, reduce heat to low, cover, and cook for 20 minutes. Remove from heat and set aside for 15 minutes.

Meanwhile, in a large frying pan, bring ½ cup (125 mL) water to a boil. Braise onions and bell peppers for 5 minutes, stirring frequently. Stir in currants and cranberries with their soaking liquid. Add herbs, ginger, almonds, green onions, cayenne pepper, and ½ tsp salt. Cook for another 5 minutes, until water is absorbed.

Remove from heat. Fluff up cooked quinoa with a fork. Stir in onion mixture. Garnish with chopped pumpkin seeds.

 "Pumpkin seeds are an excellent source of vitamins A, B, and C as well as zinc. Pumpkin seeds are being studied for their role in treating benign prostatic hyperplasia. They have traditionally been used to ease urinary ailments and expel tapeworms. In Southeastern Austria, cooks use dark green pumpkin seed oil in both green and potato salads." —Ilse

CORN & BEAN SKILLET

This wholesome and flavorful dish is a meal in itself. You may use any variety of beans you prefer and adjust the spices to taste.

MAKES 2–3 SERVINGS

Crust:

¼ tsp salt

½ cup (125 mL) coarse cornmeal

¼ tsp ground cumin

¼ tsp ground coriander seeds

1 tbsp extra virgin olive oil

In a large pot on high heat, bring 1½ cups (375 mL) water to a boil. Add ¼ tsp salt, reduce heat to medium, and slowly add cornmeal in a steady flow, stirring constantly to prevent lumps or burning. Reduce heat to low. Add cumin, coriander, and oil and simmer for 15 minutes. Spoon cornmeal into a large very lightly oiled oven-proof cast iron pan and set aside.

Topping:

1 small onion, finely chopped

1 small tomato, finely chopped or ½ cup (125 mL) finely chopped sun-dried tomatoes

½ cup (125 mL) diced yellow or red bell peppers

1 garlic clove, pressed or grated

½ tsp dried basil

½ tsp dried thyme

½ tsp Himalayan salt

½ tsp cayenne pepper, or to taste

½ cup diced carrots

1 cup (250 mL) cooked beans (such as black, pinto, or kidney)

1 cup (250 mL) fresh or frozen corn

½ cup (125 mL) finely chopped fresh cilantro, for garnish

Preheat oven to 375°F (190°C).

In a medium oven-proof frying pan on medium-high heat, braise onions in ½ cup (125 mL) water for about 5 minutes, until soft. Stir in tomatoes, bell peppers, garlic, herbs, cayenne pepper, carrots, beans and corn, and cook for 10 minutes. Spoon over crust. Bake for 15 minutes. Serve garnished with finely chopped cilantro.

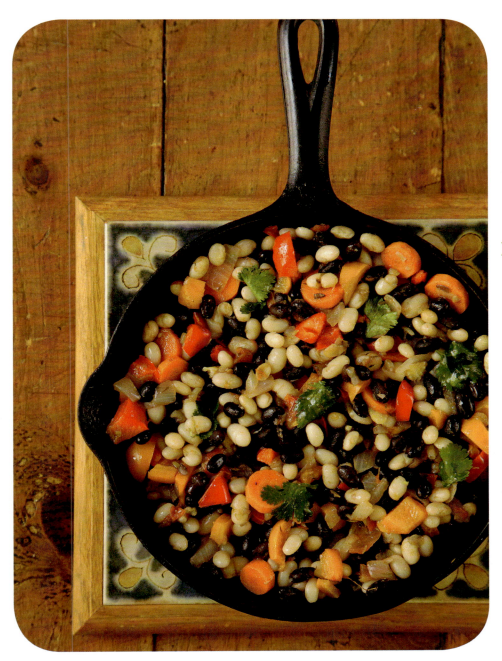

> "Cayenne is good not only for the digestive system, but also for heart and circulation. It has antifungal qualities and is helpful in preventing and treating blood clots. For external use, cayenne is made into creams, tinctures, and liniments, which ease the pain of arthritis and rheumatism. Cayenne drives away rodents and insect pests and, in ancient times, was believed to ward off vampires and werewolves. I always carry a little bottle of cayenne in my purse—just in case!" —Ilse

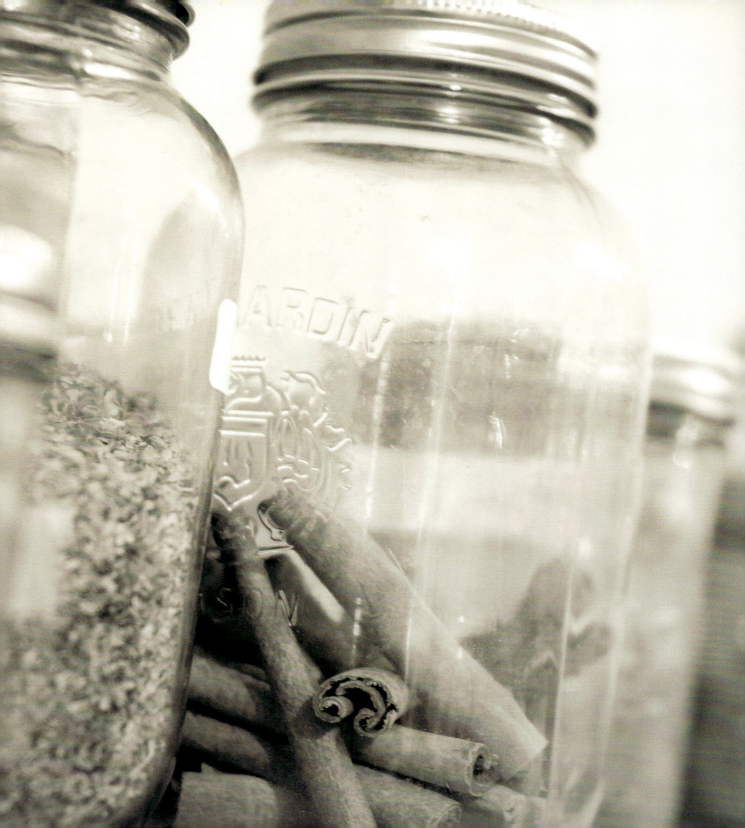

DESSERTS & SWEET TREATS

Tibetan Ants on a Log 178

Lemon Poppy Seed Energy Bites 179

Yum Rum Balls 180

Almond Dream Bars 181

Austrian Linzer Squares 182

Date Me Squares 183

Righteous Brownies with Caramel Frosting 184

Luscious Lemon Cheezecake with Strawberry Jam 186

Autumn Apple Crumble 188

Vanilla Kream 189

Praline Kream 189

Apple Kream Pie 190

Better Pecan Pie with Shortbread Crust 191

Orange Chocolate Blossom Tart 192

Cloud Lime Pie 193

Peppermint Patties 194

Black Magic 195

Chocolate Almond Butter Cups 196

Russian Kissel 198

Omi's Fruit Compote 199

Midnight Fantasy Chocolate Mousse 200

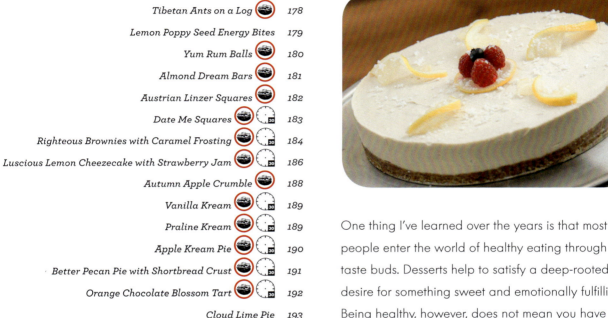

One thing I've learned over the years is that most people enter the world of healthy eating through their taste buds. Desserts help to satisfy a deep-rooted desire for something sweet and emotionally fulfilling. Being healthy, however, does not mean you have to give up sweets: everyone needs to take pleasure in a luxurious dessert once in a while.

When we think of dessert, we often think of sinfully rich indulgences created with fat, sugar, refined flours, and other unhealthy ingredients that provide a temporary high. Raw desserts are a different story. Although luscious and bold in flavor, they are made with healthy, unrefined, whole food ingredients and are free from processed products. Raw desserts never fail to impress! The following recipes are full of nutrition and flavor, and will complement any meal. Most can be made in advance and stored in the refrigerator or freezer.

Before I "came out" as a raw foodist, I would bring raw pies, cakes, or other sweet treats to family gatherings. It delighted me to observe the happy reactions of both young children and their grandparents when they tasted my raw vegan creations. Of course, they had no idea (at the time) that the decadent desserts were uncooked and actually good for them! Now, my family requests my raw desserts all the time!

▶ *All good stories have sweet endings, just like perfect meals.*

▶ *If a recipe calls for dry nuts or seeds, the best option is to soak (6–8 hours) and then dehydrate (12–24 hours), but you can use raw dry nuts instead.*

TIBETAN ANTS ON A LOG

MAKES ABOUT 30 STUFFED CELERY PIECES

Don't worry—no ants have been harmed in the making of this dish!

about 2 cups (500 mL) almond butter
1 tbsp raw tahini
2 tbsp maple syrup
¼ cup (60 mL) hot purified water
juice of 1 small orange
1 tbsp ground cardamom seeds
1 tbsp grated fresh ginger
⅛ tsp ground allspice
⅛ tsp ground coriander
cayenne pepper, to taste
10 celery stalks
½ cup (125 mL) dried goji berries soaked in ¼ cup (60 mL) orange juice for 15 minutes
1 cup (250 mL) alfalfa sprouts

In a bowl, combine almond butter, tahini, maple syrup, hot water, orange juice, cardamom, ginger, allspice, coriander, and cayenne. Cut celery stalks into 3-in (8-cm) pieces. Spread almond butter mixture on celery and arrange a line of goji berries on mixture (these are the "ants"). Arrange stalks on a large platter with sprouts.

LEMON POPPY SEED ENERGY BITES

MAKES ABOUT 20 BITE-SIZED BALLS

A zesty, nut-free treat full of delicious goodness. Make these in advance and store in the refrigerator.

1 cup (250 mL) dry sunflower seeds
1 cup (250 mL) dry pumpkin seeds
1 cup (250 mL) coconut flour
¼ tsp Himalayan salt
1 cup (250 mL) pitted Medjool dates
1 tsp vanilla extract
1 tbsp lemon zest
¼ cup (60 mL) or more lemon juice
3 tbsp poppy seeds
¼ cup (60 mL) shredded coconut

In a food processor, process sunflower and pumpkin seeds until flour-like. Add coconut flour, salt, dates, vanilla extract, lemon zest, and lemon juice and process until mixture begins to form into a ball. Add poppy seeds and process briefly. Remove from food processor and form into bite-sized balls. Roll in shredded coconut. Will keep for 2 weeks in refrigerator or 3 months in freezer.

*Goji berries, also known as Chinese wolfberries or **Lycium barbarum**, have been used in traditional Chinese medicine for hundreds of years to restore energy and strength, increase stamina and longevity, strengthen the immune system, boost sexual libido, and improve eyesight. They are a rich source of iron and zinc and vitamins A, C, and E. Buy certified organic or USDA certified. Avoid goji berries that are bright red or bright orange-red, as they may have been treated with sulfites.*

YUM RUM BALLS

MAKES ABOUT 20 RUM BALLS

My father would sometimes surprise the family with a box of rum balls and, ever since, I get nostalgic for them at Christmas. One year, while watching my mother prepare her traditional Christmas rum balls with butter for the annual cookie exchange, I was inspired to make a raw vegan version: it's tastier than the standard rum ball and is more nutritious, too.

3 cups (750 mL) dry almonds (see p. 41)
¾ cup (185 mL) maple syrup
1 cup (250 mL) raw cacao powder
1 tsp vanilla extract
⅛ tsp Himalayan salt
3 tbsp dark rum or 2 tsp rum extract
¼–½ cup (60–125 mL) cacao nibs, coarsely ground

In a food processor, process almonds until flour-like. Add ground almonds to a mixing bowl. Stir in remainder of ingredients, except ground cacao nibs, and mix to combine well. Form into bite-sized balls and roll in cacao nibs. This can get messy (especially if you dip into the rum!).

▶ *Cacao nibs are partially ground cacao beans. You can coarsely grind them further in a coffee grinder. They have a rather bitter flavor and are a healthier alternative to chocolate chips but, like other chocolate products, are stimulating (some people eat them straight out of the bag!). They can be added to smoothies and desserts. If you have extra, store in the refrigerator for up to 6 months.*

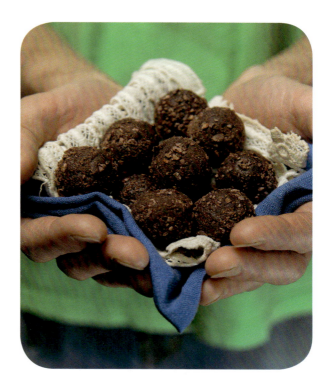

ALMOND DREAM BARS

MAKES ABOUT 12–16 SQUARES

Sweet, rich, and dreamy—this is heaven on your tongue!

Crust:

3 cups (750 mL) dry almonds

1½ cups (375 mL) pitted Medjool dates

½ cup (125 mL) cacao powder

1 tsp vanilla extract

⅛ tsp Himalayan salt

Filling:

½ cup (125 mL) + 2 tbsp almond butter

½ cup (125 mL) coconut oil

¼ cup (60 mL) packed coconut butter (p. 145)

½ cup (125 mL) + 1 tbsp maple syrup

2 tsp lucuma powder (optional)

1 tbsp vanilla extract

⅛ tsp Himalayan salt

¼ tsp ground cinnamon

In a food processor, process almonds until flour-like. Add dates, cacao, vanilla extract, and salt, blending until mixture begins to stick together. Press evenly into an 8 x 8-in (2-L) pan. Spoon filling into pan. Refrigerate for 1 hour to firm up before cutting into squares.

➤ *Although optional, using just a bit of salt in desserts really enhances the overall flavor.*

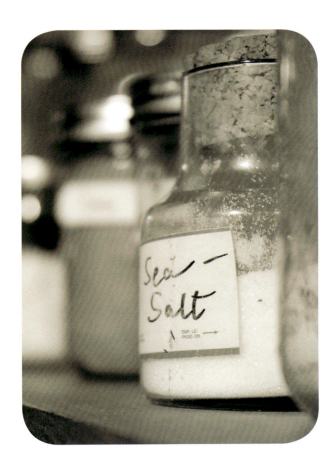

AUSTRIAN LINZER SQUARES

MAKES ABOUT 12–16 SQUARES

The Linzer Torte is named after the city of Linz, Austria, where it is often served at local *kaffeehauses* and bakeries. It is traditionally made from sugar, butter, flour, almonds, and raspberry preserves. When I first created this raw version, I hoped my Austrian mother would approve. She did! These squares are also very popular with customers at our restaurant, SimplyRaw Express.

Crust:

3 cups (750 mL) coconut flour

1 cup (250 mL) cashew flour

⅛ tsp Himalayan salt

¼ cup (60 mL) maple syrup

1 tsp vanilla extract

zest of ½ lemon

Raspberry Jam:

1 cup (250 mL) fresh or frozen raspberries (thawed)

½ cup (125 mL) pitted Medjool dates

In a food processor, blend coconut and cashew flours and salt briefly to mix. Add maple syrup, vanilla extract, and lemon zest, and blend until well combined. Evenly press ⅔ of mixture into an 8 x 8-in (2-L) pan, using the back of a spoon to flatten and set aside.

In a blender, blend raspberries and dates until smooth. Pour mixture over crust and spread evenly. Top with remainder of crust. Chill in refrigerator for at least 2 hours.

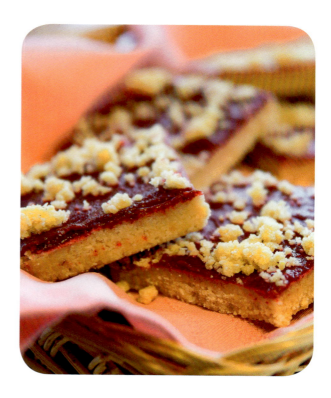

DATE ME SQUARES

MAKES ABOUT 12–16 SQUARES

I have been making this simple recipe for years, and it continues to be a favorite with friends, family, and SimplyRaw Express patrons. These are delicious, and your guests will be convinced that you've been in the kitchen baking them for hours. (Your secret's safe with me!)

 If you don't have time to first soak and dehydrate nuts, use plain raw nuts for a second-best option.

Crumble:

2 cups (500 mL) dry walnuts

1 cup (250 mL) dry almonds

½ cup (125 mL) coconut flour

¼ tsp ground cinnamon

3–4 tbsp maple syrup

dash Himalayan salt

Filling:

2 cups (500 mL) pitted Medjool dates, soaked for 30 minutes

juice and zest of ½ orange

1 cup (250 mL) dried cranberries, soaked for 30 minutes

In a food processor, process walnuts and almonds until coarsely ground. Add coconut flour, cinnamon, maple syrup, and salt and pulse until mixture begins to stick together. Evenly press ⅔ of mixture into an 8 x 8-in (2-L) pan.

In a blender or food processor, process filling ingredients until smooth. Pour over crumble mixture. Top with remainder of crumble. Refrigerate for at least 2 hours.

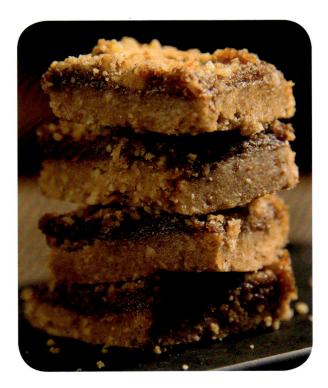

RIGHTEOUS BROWNIES WITH CARAMEL FROSTING

These brownies can be made (and devoured!) in just a matter of minutes, but they also store well in the freezer. Frosting is optional, but well worth the extra step.

MAKES ABOUT 12–16 BROWNIES

Brownies:

1 cup (250 mL) dry pecans

1 cup (250 mL) dry walnuts

1 cup (250 mL) coconut flour

⅛ tsp Himalayan salt

½ cup (125 mL) pitted Medjool dates

¾ cup (185 mL) cacao powder

2 tbsp almond butter

½ cup (125 mL) maple syrup

1 tbsp vanilla extract

In a food processor, process pecans, walnuts, coconut flour, and ⅛ tsp salt until finely ground. Add dates, cacao powder, almond butter, maple syrup, and vanilla extract and blend until well combined. Evenly press mixture into 8 x 8-in (2-L) pan.

Frosting:

1 cup (250 mL) cashews, soaked for 30 minutes or more

½ cup (125 mL) maple syrup

¼ cup (60 mL) coconut sugar

1 tbsp vanilla extract

¼ tsp Himalayan salt

1 tsp lucuma powder (optional)

¼ cup (60 mL) melted coconut oil

¼ cup (60 mL) cacao nibs, for garnish

In a blender or food processor, blend cashews, maple syrup, sugar, vanilla extract, ¼ tsp salt, and lucuma powder until smooth. Add coconut oil and blend until well combined. Spread frosting over brownies and sprinkle with cacao nibs.

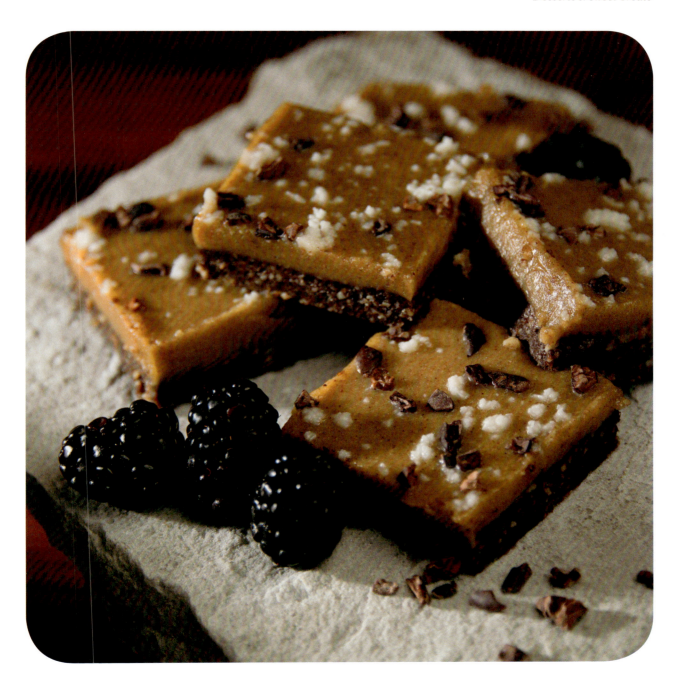

LUSCIOUS LEMON CHEEZECAKE WITH STRAWBERRY JAM

Impress your friends—whether or not they're raw foodists—with this rich and refreshing cheezecake. It can be made in advance and frozen for a few weeks. The jam is optional but provides a lovely garnish. With or without jam, this zesty cake is a winner!

MAKES 10–12 SERVINGS

Crust:

1½ cups dry almonds

dash Himalayan salt

2 tbsp shredded coconut

¼ cup (60 mL) packed, pitted Medjool dates

1 tsp vanilla extract

In a food processor, process almonds with salt until it forms a fine flour. Add remainder of crust ingredients and process until mixture starts to stick together. Press into an 8-in (20-cm) springform pan. Refrigerate while making the filling.

Filling:

3 cups (750 mL) cashews, soaked for 30 minutes or more

1 cup (250 mL) lemon juice

zest of 1 lemon

¾ cup maple syrup

1 tbsp vanilla extract

dash Himalayan salt

½ cup (125 mL) melted coconut oil

In a blender, process cashews with lemon juice, lemon zest, maple syrup, vanilla extract, and salt until smooth. Add coconut oil and blend again. Pour over crust. Refrigerate for at least 4 hours before serving. It also freezes well.

Strawberry Jam:

2 cups (500 mL) fresh or frozen strawberries

½ cup (125 mL) pitted Medjool dates

1 tsp vanilla extract

1 tbsp psyllium powder (optional)

In a blender, blend all jam ingredients until smooth. Store in a squeeze bottle and drizzle onto cheesecake or beside a slice of it on a plate.

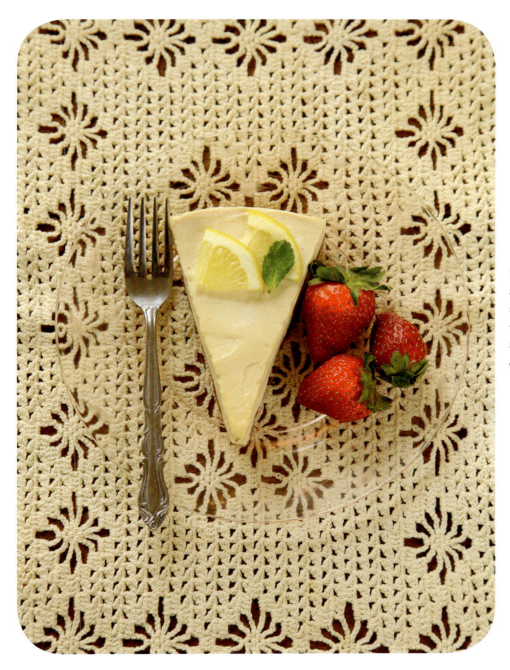

Tip: *Flip the bottom of your removable springform pan upside down before filling with crust. This will make it easier to remove the cheezecake.*

AUTUMN APPLE CRUMBLE

MAKES 6–8 SERVINGS

Is there anything more delicious than grandma's old-fashioned apple crumble? Raw apple crumble! This is a wonderfully simple yet delicious way to enjoy summer's bounty. (It can also be made from other fruits in season.) Serve topped with Vanilla Kream (opposite).

Filling:

6 large apples, peeled, cored, and finely chopped

2 tbsp lemon juice

½ cup (125 mL) Thompson raisins

¼ cup (60 mL) pitted Medjool dates

3 tbsp maple syrup

1 tsp vanilla extract

¼ tsp ground nutmeg

zest of ½ orange

1 tsp ground cinnamon

dash Himalayan salt

In a large bowl, toss 4 finely chopped apples with lemon juice and raisins. In a food processor, process remainder of ingredients until smooth. Combine with apple mixture and remaining 2 chopped apples, tossing to combine well. Transfer to an 8 x 8-in (2-L) pan or into individual serving cups or ramekins.

Topping:

½ cup (125 mL) dry walnuts

½ cup (125 mL) dry almonds

2 tbsp coconut sugar

½ cup (125 mL) coconut flour

½ cup (125 mL) pitted Medjool dates

⅛ tsp Himalayan salt

1 tsp vanilla extract

1 tsp ground cinnamon

1 tbsp coconut oil

In a food processor, pulse walnuts and almonds until coarsely ground. Add remainder of ingredients, processing until crumbly. Do not over-process or mixture will become too oily. Crumble mixture over the apples with your hands, pressing lightly. Apple Cobbler will keep for up to 3 days in the refrigerator.

VANILLA KREAM

MAKES ABOUT 1 CUP (250 mL)

This is an incredibly easy and versatile recipe that can be used to replace dairy cream. A dollop on a piece of pie or crumble creates instant luxury!

1 cup (250 mL) cashews, soaked for 30 minutes or more
¼ cup (60 mL) purified water
3 tbsp maple syrup
1 tbsp vanilla extract
1 tbsp lemon juice
3 tbsp melted coconut oil
¼ tsp Himalayan salt

In a blender, blend all ingredients until creamy. Store refrigerated in an airtight container or squeeze bottle.

PRALINE KREAM

MAKES 2–4 SERVINGS

A creamy, sweet raw vegan pudding that tastes just like butter pecan.

1 cup (250 mL) pecans, soaked for 8 hours
½ cup (125 mL) purified water
½ cup (125 mL) prepared Irish moss gel
1 tbsp vanilla extract
1 tbsp gluten-free tamari
¼ tsp Himalayan salt
¼ cup (60 mL) maple syrup
1 tsp ground cinnamon
2 tbsp melted coconut oil
2–4 dry pecans, for garnish

In a blender or food processor, blend all ingredients, except coconut oil and pecans, until smooth. Add coconut oil and blend again. Taste and adjust sweetness. Spoon into individual parfait glasses and top each with a whole pecan.

 See "Preparing Irish Moss" on p. 44.

APPLE KREAM PIE

MAKES 8–12 SERVINGS

A rich and creamy pie, delicate in flavor and full of nourishment. You'll never bake another apple pie again!

Crust:

1 cup (250 mL) dry walnuts

1 cup (250 mL) dry almonds

¼ cup (60 mL) coconut flour

½ cup (125 mL) pitted Medjool dates

1 tsp vanilla extract

dash Himalayan salt

In a food processor, process walnuts, almonds, coconut flour, and dates until mixture begins to stick together. Add vanilla extract and salt and blend again. Press into a 9-in (23-cm) deep-dish glass pie plate. Refrigerate while making filling.

Filling:

3 cups (750 mL) cored and grated apples

1 tbsp lemon juice

1 cup (250 mL) Thompson raisins

2 cups (500 mL) cashews, soaked for 30 minutes or more

½ tsp ground nutmeg

1 tsp ground cinnamon

½ tsp ground allspice

3 tbsp maple syrup

2 tbsp melted coconut oil

1 tbsp vanilla extract

1 apple, cored and thinly sliced, for garnish

In a large bowl, combine grated apples with lemon juice and raisins.

In a blender, blend remainder of ingredients with ½ cup (125 mL) purified water until smooth and creamy. Fold into apple mixture and mix well by hand. Pour over crust. Garnish top of pie with apple slices.

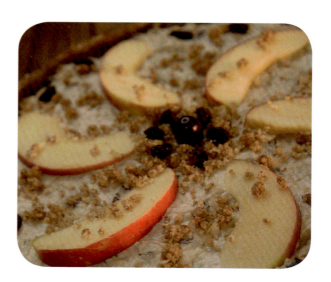

BETTER PECAN PIE WITH SHORTBREAD CRUST

MAKES ABOUT 10 SERVINGS

This is pecan pie perfection. Traditional pecan pie is so *old news!*

Shortbread Crust:

2½ cups (625 mL) coconut flour

1½ cups cashew flour

⅛ tsp Himalayan salt

3 tbsp maple syrup

1 tsp vanilla extract

1 tbsp melted coconut oil

In a food processor, process all crust ingredients until mixture begins to stick together. Evenly press into an 8-in (20-cm) glass pie plate. Use back of spoon to smooth bottom and sides. Set aside (and don't bother to wash the processor!).

Filling:

1½ cups (375 mL) pitted Medjool dates, soaked for 30 minutes

¼ cup (60 mL) maple syrup

2 cups (500 mL) pecans, soaked for 8 hours

3 tbsp melted coconut oil

2 tsp ground cinnamon

1 tbsp vanilla extract

⅛ tsp Himalayan salt

about 12 dry pecans, for garnish

In a food processor, blend dates with maple syrup. Add remainder of ingredients except pecans and blend until creamy. Add 1 tsp water at a time, if needed. Spoon mixture over crust. Refrigerate for at least 2 hours. Once chilled, cut into wedges and garnish with pecans.

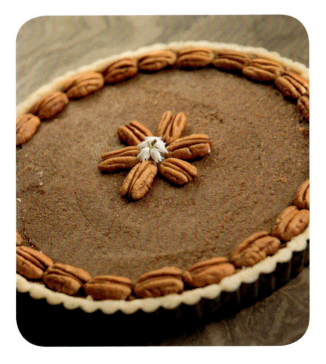

ORANGE CHOCOLATE BLOSSOM TART

MAKES 10–12 SERVINGS

A sweet and heavenly tart—guaranteed to satisfy any chocolate craving. You can use mint extract instead of orange extract for a different but equally delicious dessert.

Crust:

2½ cups (625 mL) dry walnuts

½ cup (125 mL) coconut flour

½ cup (125 mL) pitted Medjool dates

2 tbsp maple syrup

2 tsp vanilla extract

dash Himalayan salt

In a food processor, process walnuts until finely crumbled. Add remainder of crust ingredients and process until mixture begins to stick together. Evenly press into 9-in (23-cm) tart pan with a removable bottom. Refrigerate for 4 hours.

Mousse:

3 cups (750 mL) cashews, soaked for 30 minutes or more

1 cup (250 mL) purified water

¾ cup maple syrup

1 tbsp vanilla extract

2 tsp orange extract

¾ cup (185 mL) cacao powder

⅛ tsp Himalayan salt

½ cup (125 mL) melted coconut oil

1 orange, peeled and segmented, for garnish (optional)

¼ cup (60 mL) coconut flakes, for garnish (optional)

In a food processor, blend cashews and water until smooth. Add remainder of ingredients, one at a time, blending each thoroughly. Pour mixture over crust and refrigerate for at least 4 hours. Garnish with slices of oranges and coconut flakes. This tart freezes well.

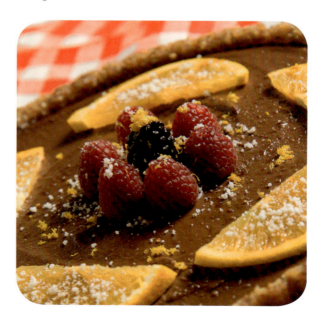

CLOUD LIME PIE

MAKES 10–12 SERVINGS

Fall in love with my all-time favorite dessert! It's nut-free and light and the perfect balance of sweet and tart. Without the crust, you can enjoy it as a pudding (as I often do) or freeze it and eat it like ice cream.

Crust:

2 cups (500 mL) coconut flour

½ cup (125 mL) packed, pitted Medjool dates

⅛ tsp Himalayan salt

1 tsp vanilla extract

2 tbsp melted coconut oil

In a food processor, process all crust ingredients until mixture begins to stick together. Add 1 tsp water, if needed. Evenly press into 8-in (20-cm) springform pan. Refrigerate while preparing the filling.

Filling:

3 ripe medium avocados

½ cup (125 mL) lime juice

¼ cup (60 mL) lemon juice

2 tbsp lime zest

½ cup (125 mL) + 1 tbsp maple syrup

½ tsp vanilla powder

⅛ tsp Himalayan salt

¼ cup (60 mL) melted coconut oil

¼ cup (60 mL) coconut butter

2 heaping tbsp prepared Irish Moss gel (optional)

1 lime, cut into thin wedges, for garnish

¼ cup (60 mL) coconut flakes, for garnish

In a food processor or blender, blend all filling ingredients, except coconut oil and butter and garnishes. Add coconut oil and butter and blend until well combined. Add Irish Moss gel, if using, and blend until just combined. Taste and adjust sweetness. Pour over crust and refrigerate for 4 hours or freeze for 1 hour. Decorate with fresh lime slices and coconut flakes.

> *If you don't have coconut butter, double up on the coconut oil instead. Adding Irish Moss will help give this filling an even fluffier, lighter texture.*

PEPPERMINT PATTIES

MAKES ABOUT 10 PATTIES

These melt-in-your-mouth chocolates taste as great as they look!

Patties:

⅓ cup (80 mL) coconut flour

⅓ cup (80 mL) cashew flour

¼ cup (60 mL) melted coconut oil

3 tbsp maple syrup

2 tsp mint extract

⅛ tsp Himalayan salt (optional)

In a blender or food processor, blend all ingredients for patties until smooth. Roll into bite-sized balls, then pat them flat (about ¼-in [6-mm] thick). Place on a platter or tray and freeze to harden, about 30 minutes.

Sauce:

3 tbsp cacao grated butter

1 tbsp melted coconut oil

¼ cup (60 mL) cacao powder

3 tbsp maple syrup

½ tsp vanilla extract

dash Himalayan salt

In a food processor, process all sauce ingredients. Transfer to a small bowl. Using a toothpick, dip each patty into the sauce. Place patties on a platter or tray and freeze until hardened, about 30 minutes.

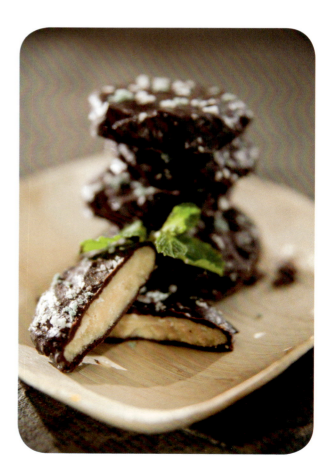

BLACK MAGIC

MAKES ABOUT 12 CHOCOLATES

This chocolate base is great for making your own healthy chocolate bars. You might have to double the recipe—it tastes so good! Experiment with optional seasonings, nuts, and dried fruits. I love to add raisins, cacao nibs, and almonds.

1 cup (250 mL) melted cacao butter

¼ cup (60 mL) melted coconut oil

¾ cup cacao powder

½ maple syrup (or to taste)

⅛ tsp Himalayan salt

2 tsp vanilla extract

about ¼ cup (60 mL) raisins (optional)

about ¼ cup (60 mL) goji berries (optional)

about ¼ cup (60 mL) almonds (optional)

about ¼ cup (60 mL) cacao nibs (optional)

about ¼ cup (60 mL) cashew pieces (optional)

2 tbsp orange, mint, or almond extract (optional)

In a bowl, combine cacao butter, coconut oil, and cacao powder and stir to combine well. Stir in maple syrup, salt, and vanilla extract, mixing well. If adding extra ingredients, stir in. Pour mixture into candy molds or ice cube trays. Freeze for about 60 minutes to harden. (If you leave at room temperature too long, it will soften and melt.)

Chocolate can be challenging to work with, so be sure to give it your full attention, with no interruptions. You'll need to work quickly and be careful not to let the chocolate overheat or allow water into the mixture, or it will curdle.

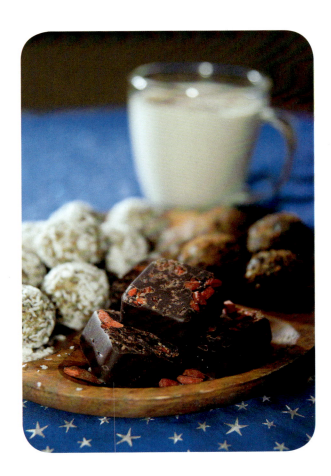

CHOCOLATE ALMOND BUTTER CUPS

A sweet treat reminiscent of peanut butter cups, but made with raw almond butter and maple syrup—a healthier alternative!

MAKES ABOUT 8 ALMOND BUTTER CUPS

Chocolate Cups:

¼ cup (60 mL) melted cacao butter

⅓ cup (80 mL) melted coconut oil

¼ cup (60 mL) maple syrup

1 tsp vanilla extract

3 tbsp cashew flour

⅓ cup (80 mL) cacao powder

⅛ tsp Himalayan salt

In a bowl, combine cacao butter, coconut oil, maple syrup, and vanilla extract. Whisk until smooth. Stir in cashew flour and cacao powder, a little at a time, until thoroughly mixed. Add ⅛ tsp salt and continue to stir for a few moments. Spoon about 1 tbsp chocolate into silicone mini-cupcake or candy molds (If you prefer a thinner cup, use less chocolate.) Freeze for about 10 minutes to harden.

Filling:

¼ cup (60 mL) almond butter

½ tsp nutritional yeast (optional)

1½ tbsp maple syrup

¼ tsp Himalayan salt

In a food processor or in a bowl by hand, combine all filling ingredients. Scoop out 1 tbsp filling at a time and roll into a ball, then flatten slightly. Place on a tray and freeze until set, about 10–15 minutes.

Remove chocolate cups and filling from freezer. Place a patty of filling in each cup. Top with remainder of chocolate sauce, using a spoon to spread it to edges. Refrigerate for about 1 hour. To remove chocolate from silicone molds, peel down and pop cups out. Store in a covered container in refrigerator or freezer.

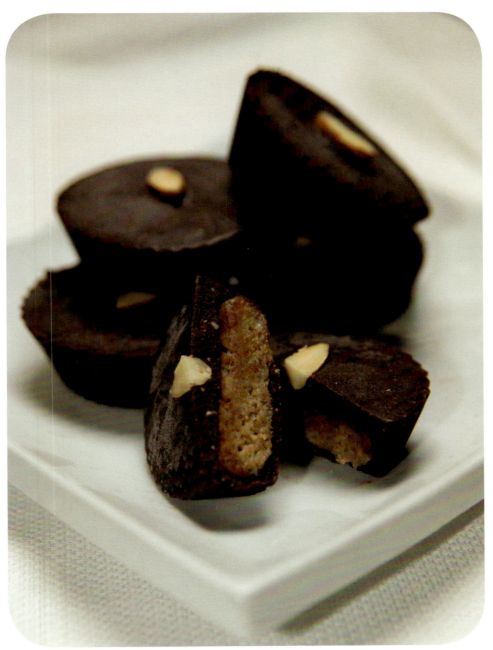

Variation: *If you are pressed for time (or lazy in the kitchen, like I can be), simply combine chocolate and almond butter mixtures in a bowl. Roll into balls and sprinkle with cacao nibs and shredded coconut. Freeze until ready to be served.*

RUSSIAN KISSEL

MAKES 4–6 SERVINGS

Kissel gets its name from the Russian word, (*kíslyj*), which means sour. This is a nutritious and refreshing dessert. Serve topped with fresh berries or slivered almonds and garnish with edible flowers or lemon balm leaves.

2 cups (500 mL) purified water

1 star anise

4 tbsp agar agar flakes, dissolved in ½ cup (125 mL) purified water

2 tbsp arrowroot powder mixed with enough water to form a paste

2 cups (500 mL) fresh or frozen raspberries

½ cup (125 mL) maple syrup

juice and zest of 1 lemon

½ tsp ground cinnamon

½ tsp ground allspice

1 tbsp freshly grated ginger

In a large pot on high heat, bring water with star anise to a boil. Slowly pour in dissolved agar agar, stirring continuously. Simmer for 5 minutes. Add arrowroot paste and boil for another 2–3 minutes. Remove from heat, discard star anise, and stir in remainder of ingredients. Whisk to evenly distribute fruit. Pour into a serving bowl or spoon into individual dishes. Set at room temperature for 90 minutes or in refrigerator for about 60 minutes.

▶ *Agar agar is a natural, colorless gelatin made from red algae. It contains calcium, iron, phosphorus, iodine, and other minerals. Used to make aspics and fruit jellies, it is a healthy, vegan alternative to gelatin, which is made from animal products.*

▶ *Native people of North America used arrowroot paste to heal wounds received from poisonous arrows—hence its name. The root is also an edible starch, from which arrowroot cookies are made.*

OMI'S FRUIT COMPOTE

MAKES 4–5 SERVINGS

My grandmother's favorite dessert was this compote, which she enjoyed both for dessert and breakfast. She lived to be 102 years old! Serve warm or cold. You may wish to add ½ cup (125 mL) wine, as Omi did.

4 large apples, cored and diced

½ cup (125 mL) maple syrup or raw sugar

6 dried apricots, halved

6 prunes, pitted and halved

⅓ cup (80 mL) dried cranberries

3 whole cloves

1 star anise

1–2 tbsp chopped fresh ginger

2-in (5-cm) length cinnamon stick

¼ cup (60 mL) lemon juice

In a large pot on high heat, bring 4 cups (1 L) purified water and all ingredients except lemon juice to a gentle boil. Simmer until apples are soft and fruit plumped, about 20 minutes. Remove cloves and star anise. Stir in lemon juice and serve warm or cold.

*Cloves are the dried flower buds of an evergreen tree, native to the Moluccas. The name comes from the French word **clou**, meaning nail or spike. Medicinally, cloves have antiseptic properties, and are chewed to soothe a sore throat. I have often used clove oil to relieve a painful toothache.*

MIDNIGHT FANTASY CHOCOLATE MOUSSE

MAKES 4 SERVINGS

Chocolate makes everything better—especially when it's made with healthy ingredients!

2 avocados, chopped

2 tbsp hemp seeds

¾ cup maple syrup

¾ cup cacao powder

2 tsp vanilla extract

1 tbsp melted coconut oil

1 tsp balsamic vinegar

½ tsp tamari

about 1 cup (250 mL) blueberries, for garnish

In a food processor, process all ingredients except garnish until smooth. Spoon into 4 glasses or bowls. Serve at room temperature or chill in refrigerator before serving. Garnish with fresh berries.

ACKNOWLEDGMENTS

I wish to express my deepest gratitude to my family:

My father Yuri, for setting the highest of expectations for me, for teaching me the morals and ethics that have made me who I am today, and for always being there for me.

My mother Ilse, who taught me the importance of healthy home cooking and who brings tremendous love and care to this world, time after time. Thank you for agreeing to contribute to this book. We should all be so active, open-minded, and flexible at eighty-five years of age!

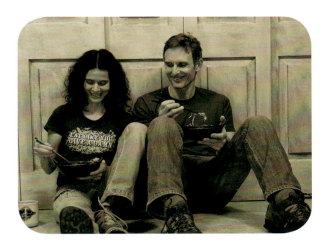

My son Mischa, the light of my life—and my number-one food critic. Thank you for understanding my long nights at the computer and for putting up with the mess in the kitchen. I can't express enough just how proud I am of you. There is no greater gift on earth than a mother's child.

My deepest love and appreciation to my husband Mark, who not only urged me to take on this project, but supported me to the very end, never allowing me to quit. *The SimplyRaw Kitchen* would not exist without your love, patience, and belief in me.

To my dear kindred friend Patricia McAllister, for reviewing and editing the early manuscript, and for our many late-night, long-distance, heart-to-heart phone calls. Here's to many, many more.

To Janet Podleski for your support, friendship, and belief in my project and vision. Your wisdom and humor is truly a breath of fresh air. Shine on.

Much gratitude to Mariel Hemingway, for touching me with your kind words and courageous life mission, and for speaking out about the difficulties of mental health and suicide. I know only too well the struggles of depression. Thank you for inspiring so many people around the world to find their best lives.

To Dr Richard Anderson for contributing the foreword to my book and for pioneering the natural health movement. Your life and work are an inspiration to millions of people—including me. Thank you for the generosity of your time and spirit. I am deeply honored.

To Dr Neal Barnard for relentlessly educating us all on the benefits of a plant-based diet. Your love for all beings touched my heart decades ago. May the world catch the wave.

To Rich Roll, whose incredible feats of athleticism show the true power and potential of a plant-based diet. Your journey to healthier living and athletic achievements are truly awe-inspiring.

I am especially grateful to Bif Naked, who embodies compassion, kindness, and strength. Your friendship and praise for my first book and support for *The SimplyRaw Kitchen* helps me believe that I am making a difference. Thank you, Biffy. You are an absolute gem.

My continuing gratitude to the entire Arsenal Pulp Press family behind this book: Brian Lam, Robert Ballantyne, Cynara Geissler, Gerilee McBride, and especially my insightful editor Susan Safyan who has now seen me through two books with unrelenting patience, professionalism, and good humor.

Many thanks to Marcia O'Hara, Amanda Borris, and Hal Walter, who offered their taste buds, support, feedback, and food-styling talents, always with enthusiasm.

A warm thank-you to Butterfly Sky Farms, for providing me with the most incredible microgreens and wheatgrass that I have ever tasted.

To my photographer Trevor Lush, for capturing the essence of not only our food, but the warm and inviting atmosphere in our kitchen.

To Breanne Gibson, who helped conduct research on this project, and was always willing to assist.

To Carolyn Best for providing The Pantry Tea Room for our first photo shoot location.

To my staff and kitchen angels at SimplyRaw Express, who continue to grow and evolve as we do. Thank you for being part of our mission to bring healthy living to the community.

I am grateful to my many wonderful clients, students, and SimplyRaw Express customers, for entrusting me with your health, and allowing me to be of service in your journey of healing and transformation.

Blessings to all of you for taking this book into your hands and for providing me with the opportunity to fulfill my passion. It is a great privilege.

INDEX

Note: Recipe titles in **bold**

agar agar, 198
agave nectar, 33
Aged Peppercorn Cheeze, 140
Airola, Paavo, 19, 24
Alkaline Mineral Broth, 93
Almond Butter & Banana Wrap, 77
Almond Dream Bars, 181
almonds, 61, 143
   butter. *See* Basic Almond Butter
   flour. *See* Easy Homemade Almond Flour
aminos, 149
Anderson, Dr Richard, 9–10, 19
Anti-Ulcer Cocktail, 55
apple crumble. *See* Autumn Apple Crumble
Apple Kream Pie, 190
appliances, kitchen. *See* kitchen tools
arrowroot, 198
Asian Pâté, 129
Austrian Blaukraut, 126
Austrian food, 15–16, 75, 114, 117, 125–26, 167–69, 172, 182
Austrian Linzer Squares, 182
Autumn Apple Crumble, 188
Avocado Dill Dressing, 124
avocados, 124, 131
Award-Winning Marinated Kale Salad, 116

Babuschka's Borscht, 98

Baby Greens with Sweet Miso Dressing, 108
bananas, 29
   freezing, 43–44
Basic Almond Butter, 142
Basic Fermented Cheeze, 138
basil, 29, 122
Basil Balsamic Dressing, 122
Basic Nut or Seed Mylk, 60
beets, 107
Better Pecan Pie with Shortbread Crust, 191
beverages, recipes, 49–69
Bircher's Raw Muesli, 75
Black Magic (chocolates), 195
blenders, 35
blending and juicing, 49–50
Bombay Kale, 115
books, recommended, 25
breakfast, 71–79
brownies. *See* Righteous Brownies
buckwheat, 74
   soaking, 39
cabbage, 55, 171
cacao butter, 69
cacao nibs, 180
cacao powder, 60
cancer, treatment of, 9–10
canned foods, 64
capsaicin, 91
Caramel Frosting, 184
caraway seeds, 168

carob, 74
cashews, 69
Cauliflower Chowder, 100
cayenne pepper, 175
celery, 93
Celery Powder, 44
Chai Mylk, 63
cheezes, 127, 136–40
chestnuts, 126
chia seeds, 31–32, 66
   soaking, 39
Chili Sauce, 164
Chili Sin Carne, 164
China Study, The (T. Colin Campbell), 17, 24, 40, 136
chipotle peppers, 161
chives, 29
Choc-O-Love Shake, 60
chocolate, 195
Chocolate Almond Butter Cups, 196
Chocolate Mylk, 63
Chocolate Tapioca, 74
Christopher, Dr John, 9
cilantro, 30
Cilantro Lime Dressing, 112
Cinnamon Mylk, 63
Cloud Lime Pie, 193
cloves, 199
coconut
   butter. *See* Homemade Coconut Butter

Coconut Flour, 42
mylk. *See* Do-It-Yourself Coconut Mylk
oil, 32
palm sugar or nectar, 32
Thai, 65
water, 65
coffee grinders, 35
cooked foods
   in transition to raw diet, 11, 18–20, 38
   recipes for, 67, 79, 93–95, 97–101, 103, 124–26, 166–74, 198–99
corn, 88
Corn & Bean Skillet, 174
Creamy Peppercorn Dressing, 123
Creamy Tahini Dressing, 109
Creamy Zucchini Bisque, 92
Crispy Romaine & Beets with Garlic Dressing, 107

dairy foods, 40–41
Dandelion & Potato Salad, 125
dandelions, 125
Date Me Squares, 183
dates and paste, 32, 43
dehydrators, 35
desserts, 177–200
dill, 30, 99
dips, 127, 130–31, 132–34
Do-It-Yourself Coconut Mylk, 64
Dragon Dipping Sauce, 150
dressings, salad, 106, 107–12, 115–24
dulse, 128

Easy Homemade Almond Flour, 41–42

Environmental Working Group, 27
exercise, health benefits of, 22

fermenting, 138
Five-Minute Guacamole, 131
flavors, balancing, 45–46
food processors, 35
Frugal Rice Salad, 124
fruit
   drying and ripening, 42–43

Garden Salad in a Jar, 111
Garden Salad with Creamy Tahini Dressing, 109
garlic, 30, 96
Garlic Dressing, 107
garlic powder, 133
genetically engineered or modified foods, 27
Get Up & Goji Cereal, 76
ginger, 30, 53
Ginger Tamari Dipping Sauce, 149
gluten-free foods, 28
goji berries, 78, 179
grains and legumes, soaking, 38
Green Curry Soup, 90
green drinks, 51–53, 56, 58–60

Happy Hemp Pesto with Parsnip Noodles, 152
hemp seeds, 64
herbs, dried and fresh, 29–31, 83
Himalayan salt. *See* salt, Himalayan
Hippocrates Health Institute, 16
Holiday Nut Nog, 68
Homemade Coconut Butter, 145
Homemade Tahini, 145

honey, 32

Incan Pilaf, 173
Inflammation Buster (beverage), 53
inflammation, treating, 55
Instant Breakfast Cereal, 76
Instant Hemp Mylk, 64
Irish moss, 44, 120
Italian Basil Tapenade, 130

Jensen, Dr Bernard, 9
Jerusalem artichokes, 51
juicers, 35
juicing. *See* blending and juicing

kaffir lime leaves, 84
kale, 113
Kelly, Dr William, 9
Kick Acid (beverage), 52
kitchen tools, 33–36
   electrical appliances, 35–36. *See also* individual appliances, e.g., blenders, dehydrators, etc.
Krautfleckerl, 168
Kreamy Alfredo with Sweet Potato Noodles, 153
Kyssa House Dressing, 122
Kyssa, Ilse, 11–12, 15–16, 30, 41, 96, 98, 117, 122, 125, 167–68, 172–73, 175

Lemon Dill Cheeze, 137
Lemon Poppy Seed Energy Bites, 179
Lentil Soup with Kale, 101
Light Garden Blend (soup), 83
Liquid Gold (beverage), 52

Live It Up Sushi with Ginger Tamari Dipping Sauce, 148–49
Living Mango Pudding, 77
locally grown foods, 18, 27–28
Lovage Dumplings, 169
lucuma powder, 33
Luscious Lemon Cheezecake with Strawberry Jam, 186

maca, 60
Macro Miso Spread, 132
main dishes, 147–75
Mango Lassi, 58
maple syrup, 33
Mason jar salads, 110–12
meat-eating, health effects, 10
Midnight Fantasy Chocolate Mousse, 200
milk. *See* mylks
mindful eating, 22
mint, 30
miso, 102, 132
Miso Soup with Shiitake Mushrooms, 103
muesli, 75
mulberries, 78
Mushroom Goulash (Gulyas), 167
mushrooms, shiitake, 103
My Daily Greens (beverage), 51
My Thai Smoothie, 56
mylks, 39–41, 60–64, 66

noodles
  kelp, 157
  parsnip, 152
  sweet potato, 153
  zucchini, 154–56. *See also* pastas, vegetable

nori, 149
nut mylk bags, 35, 40
nutritional yeast, 152
nuts and seeds, 31–32
  butter, 41
  fermenting, 138
  flour, 41–42
  mylk, 39–40, 60–64, 66
  soaking, 37–39

oils, 106
  cooking with, 36
Omi's Fruit Compote, 199
One-Minute Miracle Mylk, 61
onion powder, 133
onions, 131, 167
Orange Chocolate Blossom Tart, 192
oregano, 30
organic foods, 26–27
Over-the-Top Taco Salad in a Jar, 112

Pantry restaurant, The, 15
parsley, 31, 166
Parsnip Noodles, 152
Pasta Primavera, 154–55
pastas, vegetable, 36–37. *See also* noodles
pâtés, 127–29
Peace & Love Porridge, 74
peanuts, 31
pecans, 61
Peppermint Patties, 194
phytochemicals, health effects, 19
Pico de Gallo, 131
pie crusts, 186, 190, 191–93
Pine Nut Parma, 142

pine nuts, 137
plant-based diet, 17–18, 23–25. *See also* vegan diet; whole foods diet
Polenta Squares, 172
Popeye Soup, 85
Potluck Surprise Slaw, 117
Praline Kream, 189
Pretty in Pink Tapioca, 73
protein, nutritional need for, 24–25
psyllium, 159
pumpkin seed oil, 117
pumpkin seeds, 173

quinoa, 173

Rad Pad Thai, 156
Raspberry Jam, 182
raw food diet, 17–22, 26. *See also* whole foods diet, vegan diet
  and children, 21
  and social occasions, 21
  community for, 21–22
  techniques, 36–46
  transition to, 17–22
Raw Man's Quiche, 158–59
Real Tomato Soup, 86
rice cookers, 36
rice, wild, 118
Righteous Brownies with Caramel Frosting, 184
Risi Bisi, 166
Romanian Cabbage Rolls, 170–71
rosemary, 31
Russian Kissel, 198
Rustic Rawtella, 144

sage, 31, 172

salad dressings. *See* dressings, salad
salads, 105–21, 124–26
salt, Himalayan, 92
sauerkraut, 114
seaweed. *See* nori; dulse; Irish moss
sesame seeds, 145
Shamrock Mint Chip Shake, 59
Shortbread Crust, 191. *See also*
    pie crusts
Simple Cashew Pine Nut
    Cheeze, 137
SimplyRaw Living Foods Detox Manual,
    138
smoothies, 56–58
soaking. *See* buckwheat, soaking;
    chia seeds, soaking; grains and
    legumes, soaking; nuts and seeds,
    soaking
Soft Taco Verde, 162
Soup Stock, 94
soups, 81–103
Sour Kream, 132
Sour Kream & Onion Dip, 133
soy products, 102
Spiced Chia Tapioca, 72
spicy foods, 161
Spicy Mexican Lime Soup, 91
Spicy Thai Salad, 120
spinach, 85
Spinach & Mushroom Dip, 134
spreads, 127, 132, 142–45
Spring Pea Pâté, 129

Standard American Diet, 10
stevia, 33
Stovetop Rice Pudding, 79
Strawberry Fields Smoothie, 57
Strawberry Jam, 186
Sugar-Kissed Pecan Mylk, 61
Sun Tea, 68
Super Natural Kale (salad), 114
Sweet Corn Chowder, 88
Sweet Green Monster
    (beverage), 56
Sweet Miso Dressing, 108
Sweet Mustard Dressing, 123
Sweet Potato Noodles, 153
sweeteners, 32–33
symbols used in book, key to, 47

tahini. *See* Homemade Tahini
tamari, 86
tea, 67–68
Thai Coconut Curried
    Vegetables, 160
Thom Kha Soup, 84
thyme, 31
Tibetan Ants on a Log, 178
tomato soup. *See* Real Tomato Soup
Tomato-Millet Soup, 97
tomatoes, 130
tools, kitchen. *See* kitchen tools
Trail Blazer's Mix, 78
Tropical Mint Smoothie, 58
TuNO Pâté, 128

turmeric, 90, 160

Vanilla Almond Mylk, 62–63
Vanilla Bean Bubble Mylk, 66
vanilla extract, 63
Vanilla Kream, 189
vanilla powder, 68
vegan diet, 17–22. *See also* plant-
    based diet; whole foods diet
vegetables, massaging, 159
Vietnamese Salad Rolls with
    Dragon Dipping Sauce, 150
vinegar, 106
Walker, Norman, 19
Warmed White Chocolate, 69
Watermelon Cooler, 54
websites, vegan athletes, 25
wheatgrass, 52
whole foods diet, 17–22, 26. *See also*
    plant-based diet; vegan diet
Wigmore, Ann, 19, 33, 114
Wild About Rice Salad, 118
Wild Garlic (or Leek) Soup, 95
wild plants, harvesting, 125

Yogi Tea, 67
Yum Rum Balls, 180

zucchini noodles. *See* noodles,
    zucchini

NATASHA KYSSA

Natasha Kyssa has been following a raw vegan life-style since 1990. She is a former international fashion model and TEDx speaker, and now runs SimplyRaw, a healthy lifestyles consulting company, and SimplyRaw Express, a vegan restaurant in Ottawa, Ontario, Canada. Her first book, *The SimplyRaw Living Foods Detox Manual*, was published by Arsenal Pulp Press in 2009. *simplyraw.ca*

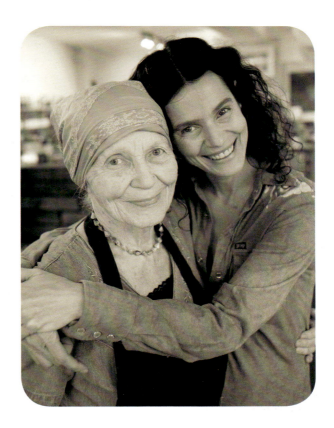